DIET and ME

DIET and ME

DR SONALI SARNOBAT

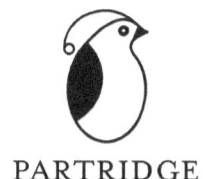

PARTRIDGE

To order additional copies of this book, contact
Partridge India
000 800 10062 62
orders.india@partridgepublishing.com

www.partridgepublishing.com/india

CONTENTS

AUTHOR'S NOTE

It is always a big question mark when it comes to weight loss and diet. Being a doctor myself makes me prone to all questions being asked. Trends change so fast that sometimes the dieticians and trainers are in a fix to judge a good diet and bad diet, likewise workout fads.

This book, though it has a lot of medical and scientific jargaon in it, readers please read it thoroughly if you really want to know the fundamentals of fitness, weightloss and diet.

Fad is always a fad but science is an ultimate truth. Follow the path of science, train yourself to accept the facts and you can easily master it.

So let's begin!

BODY BASICS

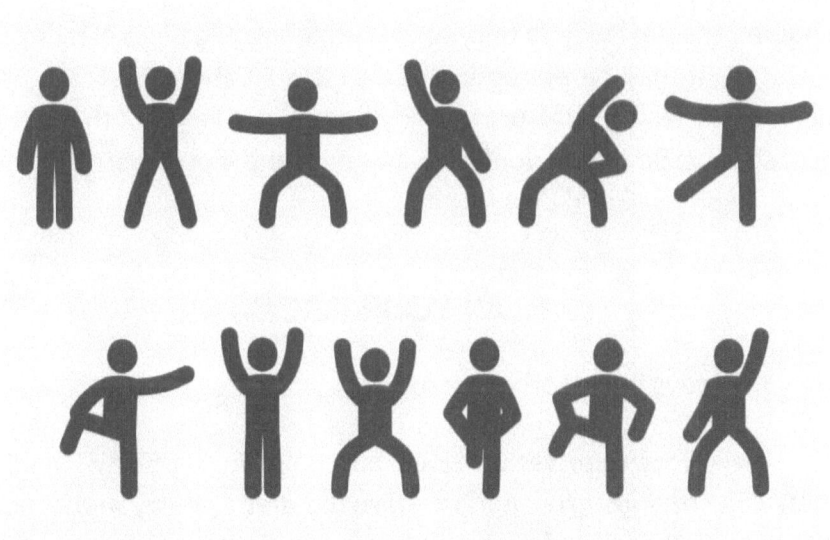

You have to understand one thing – we're not actors who roam about with their personal chefs who cook us personalised high protein meals! We don't even have a lot of money to spend on all sorts of pre-workouts, fat burners, casein, hydro-whey, and that high-end expensive stuff. I, myself, was an ordinary middle class wife and a mother, who worked. So, there is none of those luxuries that glamour brings, neither do you need any of that. We learn to do the best with whatever we have available in our budget.

Before getting to it, please understand a few things very clearly:

1. **Fitness is science**. If you're getting desired results without needing a proper plan for nutrition and workout, then good for you, you can stop reading this document right away.
2. To lose weight, you have to take lesser calories than your **Total Daily Energy Expenditure (TDEE)*,** to gain weight you have to take more calories than that. Simple and logical.

That's it, and there is absolutely NO WAY around these two guidelines. Let science guide your transformation journey, not bro-science.

I figured the best way to tell you everything would be to start from the start. It may be boring initially, as it is all about basic science behind our health, but trust me, you'll see almost 99% of the things are relevant. So please don't skip anything and if possible re-read it multiple times. Good Luck!

KNOW YOUR FOOD

Do you always feel deprived of food?

The feeling of deprivation does not help in sustained weight loss. *The cravings after a long depriving diet are way more than they are on a well-balanced diet.* If you cannot master the art of moderation in your life (in terms of your eating habits) the vicious cycle of weight gain and loss will always haunt you. **Find foods that you really like and try to add them to your diet. This could be something as simple as some rice every night for dinner.** This will not only make you feel satisfied but also will help you maintain your sanity with your overall dieting efforts. Depriving yourself of a particular food item in order to achieve your goals is never the right thing to do.

Is your diet too rigid?

There is a fine line between what usually people think about "flexible dieting" versus actually having a certain level of flexibility in your diet. If your diet is flexible enough to help you make good choices and helps you stick as closely as possible to your calorie and macro nutrient intake goal, then there is no reason why you cannot follow a flexible approach. **As long as you are getting 80% of your daily calories from whole and nutritious foods, and being flexible the remaining 20% just helps you adhere to your diet better, then you have already won the battle. Remember what helps you stick to the diet is what it all comes down to, because no macro spilt, no calorie goal, no killer workout plans will help you until you master the art of adherence.** Bring in flexibility to your diet to reap better benefits.

Do you miss out important events in your life because of your diet?

It has been 6 months that you have been dieting and you still always fear going to a party just because you will miss out on your diet and workout. You do not like entertaining guests at home, neither do you like attending gatherings of even close family members – again for the same reason. If that's the case, then you are just ruining your social life for nothing. Always remember, a bad day does not mean you will lose all your progress that you have made so far, or that you will gain all that weight that you had lost with months of effort. The scale might fluctuate a bit after a night of eating out, but that also means there is more water and sodium retention due to the diet deviation. But *how much* does it matter? *As long as you are getting back to track the next day, this barely makes any difference.* The real deal is to not stop because you had a bad day but to get back and continue your health and fitness journey, because always remember; it is You vs You!

Is your quality of life being affected due to your diet?

If you are feeling any of the above or anything even beyond that, if you are constantly being stressed out because of your diet and if you always feel fatigued and tired, then stop doing what you are currently doing, and revisit your diet and workout plans. **Your fitness journey should be a manifesto of a healthy and fit lifestyle. You should feel active and energetic and feel good about the entire process. This will not only bring a positive impact on achieving your goals but also help prevent negative signals from hitting your brain.** Remember the brain always senses the negative signals as a threat and opposes everything your body is trying to do. So, if you want the brain to be in sync with your body goals, send the right signals. Be happy about the journey and enjoy the process, it will make your life so much better, and improve the quality of life. After all that is all that really matters.

So if you are still trying to figure out the right way to balance your dieting efforts with your life in general, try getting to the bottom of these questions and resolving the underlying concerns. You will find that achieving your fitness goals is actually easier than ever.

WHY DO I FEEL HUNGRY?

Well, energy is clearly spent when you do physical work but as it turns out, a vast majority work is latent – it happens anyhow without you noticing it. This energy expenditure is measured by what is called the **Basic Metabolic Rate (BMR)**, and trust me, it is a LOT.

To take an example, the body spends energy on pumping your blood around, to different stations. Every hour, about 80 litres of blood pass through your kidneys. Furthermore, the body needs to do work to keep you warm enough. And then there is the brain, which always requires a lot of energy to keep background processes running, even if you are not actively 'thinking'.

You'll be surprised to know that our 'active' functions (doing things) actually requires much less energy as compared to the BMR. However, you can easily, raise your BMR by exercising – while the exercise itself does not really cost a lot of energy, the bodily infrastructure created for it will.

The body does not always expend energy the same way and in the same amounts.

This has everything to do with strategy.

The body's strategy in general, appears to be a lot like a modern laptop: to go on as long as possible with the available fuel. Such a strategy boils down to spending a lot of energy when it is abundant, and powering down (battery conservation mode) in its (perceived) absence. It also means whining for more energy even when a lot is available, just like a laptop claiming that its battery has run out when in fact it has hours left!

True, the body appears to have quite in attitude! As mentioned before, most healthy adults carry enough energy with them to survive at least a month. Most of us, in fact, carry around considerably more. While 'surviving' sounds big, here is what it really means – it could probably be safely said that not eating for a whole week would not even tax the prowess of our metabolism.

Yet after skipping lunch, you will probably feel starved by the time you eat dinner.

How come?

Well, it's a strategy. The body appears much attached to its energy stores. So attached, that most of us eat blindly well above our required caloric levels, and grow blissfully overweight – yet still feel hungry if we miss a single meal!

Strategy in detail – The strategy employed determines how energy is spent in the body, and how a demand for more is created. The demand part is easy. Whenever the body runs short of one kind of fuel, it sends unmistakable signals that you should eat, even though it could also deal with the situation by conversion of another plentiful source into energy. Talk about greed!

Regarding energy expenditure, the human body is generally described to be in any of these three states at any point in time: fed, fasting, or starved.

The **'Fed State'** starts sometime after eating and continues for a number of hours, after which the metabolism is said to be in the **'fasting'** state. When asleep at night, for instance, the body is fasting. (which is why we take 'break-fast'.) **Starvation** only occurs when eating does not occur for an extended period of time.

Now, when food has not arrived for a while, the body starts conserving energy in preparation of perceived hard times ahead. There are a lot of ways to do so-lowering the body temperature a bit, neglecting body maintenance, slowing down the brain etc.

This was about Food and Energy, and it was important for you to know.

We've been discussing food for so long now, aren't you wondering where water comes into picture?

ROLE OF WATER

Let's start with discussing blood. The blood serves as a medium for taking fuel to the cells, but it also works to transport away stuff the cells have discarded. What this means is, if left uncleansed of these waste products, the bloodstream would quickly become polluted. So, there are at least three organs working on cleaning it up: the two kidneys and the liver.

The kidneys function primarily as sophisticated filters. As long as things are kept wet enough, they are able to romove waste from the blood by osmosis. This waste may be further treated, and is eventually sent to the bladder for excretion out of the body.

The liver is a much more complex organ capable of advanced –level functions. It actually converts a lot of waste products into usable substances again. It can also break down molecules which cannot be filtered by the kidneys. Almost all energy conversions taking place in your body are centred around the liver.

The kidneys primarily need water to function – they need to be wetter than your blood. If they cease to be so, they become unable to filter the waste-laden blood, leaving (part of) this job to the liver. The liver then becomes occupied doing that and has less time or capacity left for conversions. When this occurs, the blood may actually enter a 'starvation' state. The liver is unable to furnish the brain with sugar and no other energy sources are available. This quickly leads to dizzy spells and general incompetence.

Effectively, what this indicates is the overwhelming importance of staying hydrated. Water is a brilliant blessing to our body, although most of us seldom realize its importance. **Staying hydrated has tremendous health benefits**. Not just for your skin, or your metabolism, or your digestion, but for optimal functioning of vital body processes.

CONCLUSIONS

All good things come to those who wait. And you have been a patient reader all this while, so this is the movement you've been waiting for. All the science we have discussed is no good if we cannot put it to some good use for our own benefit. Here are few pointers i would like to state outright;

In order *to lose Weight*, we must make sure that the following conditions are met;

- Energy intake must be decreased from maintenances levels, and energy has to be used *and not stored* in. the body.
- Energy use must not be diminished at any time, rather it should be increased through efforts.
- Stored fuels should be able to deliver the missing energy that the body needs.
- The body is a simple container – to lose weight, more energy must be expended
- Than is added. If done wrong, eating severely less (starving yourself) will actually gain you weight in the long run!
- Drinking plenty of water will actually allow liver to do the conversions and burn fat, so if u look at it this way, drinking more water does help burn fat.

I have divided the book into three main parts, nutrition, training and supplements. I wil discuss nutrition first, then training, finally followed by supplements in the order of their importance.

METABOLISM

Your body is like a car – it needs fuel to run. However, unlike a petrol or diesel car, your body can use multiple fuels. In simple word, the process in which your body uses the fuel to provide energy to your body is called **Metabolism**.

Food contains ingredients which your body can use as fuel. But even this fuel is not yet in the form of an energy that can be used immediately! If I give you a fully charged battery, try using it to bake an egg. Possible? No.

Having an energy containing fuel does not mean that is ready to use.

It all starts with food, and its **Metabolically Active Ingredients** –
- **Fat**
- **Fiber**
- **Long carbohydrates**
- **Short carbohydrates** (sugar in other words)
- **Protein**

Fat contains 9 calories (kilocalories) per gram, and carbohydrates and protein contain 4 calorie per gram each. While fibers do contains about 2 kcals, they are extremely important in making digested food leave your body. They help in digestion as well. Here's a simpler presentation;

1g of Fat = 9 calories
1g of carbohrydates = 4 calories
1g of protein = 4 calories

So far, we have discussed the fuel sources, but what exactly are these fuels that we've been talking about? What do they comprise of?

Let's have a look; -

Your body can extract at least the following three kinds of fuel from What you ingest;
1. Free fatty acids 5. Fibers (used for excreting ingredients)
2. Glucose 6. Long carbohydrates -> shorter -> glucose
3. Amino acids 7. Shorter carbohydrates ('sugars') -> glucose
4. Fat -> Free Fatty Acids 8. Proteins -> Amino Acids

Now that we know what the actual fuels are, it's time to understand how they are stored in the body. Different kinds of fuels are stored in different forms and different amounts, and in different locations.

1. FATTY ACIDS

Almost any cell can store fatty acids, they can also be transported directly in the bloodstream – no conversion is needed. If it turns out that you do not have enough cells to store all fatty acids, your body can easily generates special, **'adipocytes'** (fat cells), which put together, form the so called **'adipose tissue'**.

As can easily be observed, the body easily stores tens of kilos of fat. As each kilo of fat can power an individual for many days, an average person actually carries enough energy in form of fat to survive for a month. An over weight person often carries enough fuel to survive for many months!

But hey! All this dosen't make fat bad. Just remember, you can survive without carbs, but without essential fats, your brain will simply stop working. So never ever cut down fat completely from your diet. You need essential fats every single day for your survival!

2. GLUCOSE

Glucose is a very small molecule and easily travels from cell to cell. This make it easily transportable. This mobility is not very well suited for actually storing sugars, so for storage, sugars are converted to glycogen. Glycogen is a molecule which consists of smaller glucoses. This size and aggregation makes it easier to store glucose.

As glycogen, sugar is stored in the liver and in muscles. Both liver and muscles can convert glucose to glycogen. The liver can convert glycogen back to glucose but muscles cannot. Muscles can however use glycogen directly if needed, or release it into the bloodstream.

What is very notable, is the limited amount of sugars which can be actually stored. Ingested glucose and small carbohydrates like table sugar travel nearly directly to the blood stream while this allows the body to rapidly utilize ingested sugar, what this eventually means is that the amount of glucose allowable in blood can be easily exceeded.

People of average weight will generally have in the order of 5 grams of glucose in their blood at any specific time. Levels above 10 grams are considered too high.

This means that a regular candybar, which contains approximately 30 grams of sugar, actually poses a great challenge to the body.

When glucose arrives (via the food we eat) in excess of 10 grams, the body releases insulin, which instructs the liver and muscles to absorb glucose from the blood. Furthermore, all parts of your body which can run on glucose start doing so as well. Consequently, the burning of fatty acids for energy production is reduced.

Beyond the bloodstream, the body can store a hundred grams of glucose. Amounts differ with the actual body mass and the physical condition of each individual body, but is generally in the order of approximately 150 grams. The glucose storage can generally be depleted in a single day, making it a very short-term fuel.

Complex carbohydrates cannot be transferred directly to the bloodstream and must be converted first, which can take quite some time. This is actually a good thing, because this delay ensures that the blood isn't overflooded with glucose.

3. PROTIENS AND AMINO ACIDS

These are found throughout the body, either bunched up as proteins or freely available amino acids. They are the building blocks and can be used to form muscle fibres, or cells, or lots of other things, all of which can also be broken down again into proteins or even amino acids. It is a reversible process. Proteins are broken down into amino acids in the intestine and then brought to the liver, where they are partly reassembled and partly released into the bloodstream.

Compared to glucose, a lot of protein is available for use at any one time. The blood alone will contain in the order of approximately 100 grams.

Compared to either glucose or fatty acids, amino acids also have *huge* uses. It can also be stated that you are a big aggregation of amino acids! They make up your DNA and mostly everything else that is interesting in your body. I know it's all so scientific, and you're waiting to get to the part where all the 'real' action begins (the info that you can get your hands dirty with), but hold your horses for that! Whatever actionable items will come, comes precisely out of this scientific information and is built on this information alone. So, don't do the mistake of skipping these facts and figures! Keep reading.

THE ACTUAL ENERGY

Now, you have the petrol ready in the storage tank, but is that enough for your car to start? Certainly not. You'll have to trigger the start button, and that is when the petrol combines with air and is ignited in the combustion chamber, resulting in the release of a short burst of very powerful energy which will drive the pistons. In case of body, this energy is called **ATP (Adenosine Tri-Phosphate)**

As I mentioned earlier, your body stores its energy in the form of the three different fuels. To be used, these fuels must each be converted to ATP. This can be done in lots of places.

Glucose - Glucose, stored in the form of glycogen, can be converted into ATP by all cells containing mitochondria, which is the power producing unit of the cell. Nearly all cells have mitochondria, which means nearly all cells can convert glucose into ATP. Muscles can even burn glycogen directly, without needing to convert it first into glucose.

Fatty acids - Pretty much the same goes for site of metabolism of fatty acids, with the very notable exception of the brain. Fatty acids cannot cross the barrier into brain cells.

The brain, however, uses loads and loads of energy in the form of glucose.

Fatty acids, however, can be converted to ketones, which can partly power the brain. But only partly. It still needs glucose, and that glucose can come from protein breakdown (from your diet, or if you do not ingest enough protein, then by breaking down the muscles)

Amino acids - Can be converted by the liver into glucose, or even into fatty acids.

Almost everything can be converted to everything else in the body. But not always and not everywhere. Important conversions are:

(A) From Glucose to Glycogen to Stored Fat

As mentioned earlier, this is done when your sugar intake has exceeded the storage capacity. This happens a lot.

(B) From Stored Fat to Glucose

Creating glucose from non-glucose parts is called **Gluconeogenesis** and this is very important. It helps power the brain using long-term energy storage (fat)

Yes, That's all you need to know about fuels and storage for now. But, the interesting stuff is yet to come. Before we go there, don't you also want to know where and how all this ATP or energy is used in the body? And what about why you feel hungry even though your body has a lot of stored fat in it?

NUTRITION

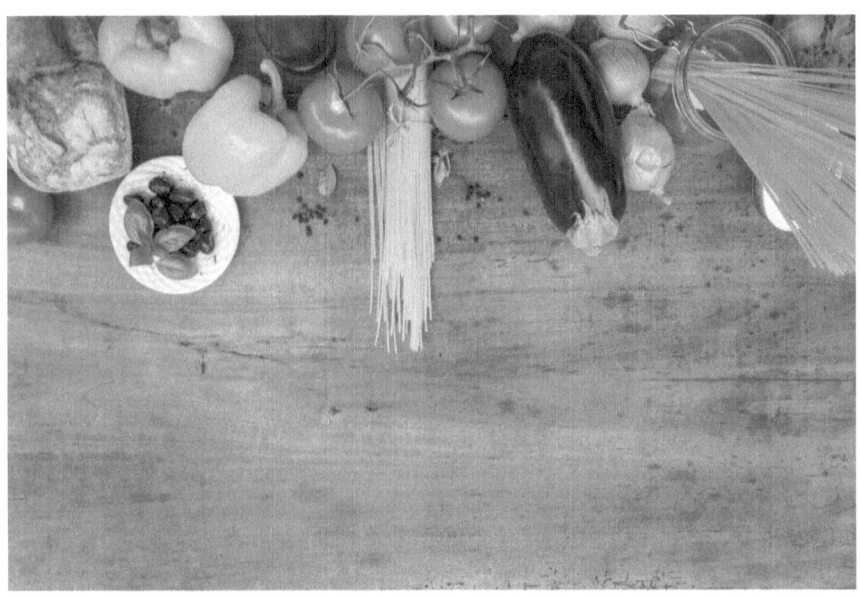

Hard work in the gym isn't something uncommon. Everyone works really hard, and yet they don't get results. I'll share my personal experience with one of my clients. When he first came to me, he was working out for two years and had an okayish physique, stomach was flat though, and definition was lacking. He was at around 12% body fat with a muscle mass of around 41 kg. After 4 weeks of following my diet, he was at 8% body fat and muscle mass of 43 kgs and he could see his abs. What changed? Diet, my friends, diet!

(I do not heavily rely upon these above mentioned statistics. I use them just for reference and so should you because the machines that check your body composition are never 100% accurate)To start with, you have to know your basal metabolic rate (BMR) or your resting metabolism.

CALCULATING THE BMR

First things first, you need to calculate your BMR, I hope you know why we're doing this? If not, please go back and read it again. However, here's the formula, on paper:

ENGLISH BMR FORMULA:
   Women BMR = 65.5+(4.35*Weight) + (4.7*Height)-(4.7*Age)
   Men BMR = 66+(6.23*Weight)+(12.7*Height)-(6.8*Age)
   Weight in Pounds, Height in Inches, Age in Years

METRIC BMR FORMULA:
   Women BMR = 65.5+(9.6*Weight)+(1.8*Height)-(4.7*Age)
   Men BMR = 66+(13.7*Weight) + (5*Height)-(6.8*Age)
   Weight in Kilograms, Height in Centimetres, Age in Years

Once you know your BMR, you can calculate your **Daily Calorie Needs** based on your activity level using the **Harris-Benedict Equation.**

To determine your total daily calorie needs, multiply your BMR by the appropriate activity factor, as follows:

Calorie-Calculation

For sedentary (little or no exercise)
=BMR*1.2
For lightly active (light exercise/sports 1-3 days/week)
=BMR*1.375

For moderately active (moderate exercise/sports 3-5 days/week)
=BMR*1.55
For very active (hard exercise/sports 6-7days a week)
=BMR*1.725

TOTAL CALORIE NEEDS EXAMPLE

If you are sedentary, multiply your BMR (1745)by 1.2=2094. This is the total number of calories you need in order to maintain your current weight.

Once you know the number of calories needed to maintain your weight, you can easily calculate the number of calories you need to eat in order to gain or lose weight.

Since our goal is to get shredded, we'll have to reduce our calorie intake. Those looking to gain weight can follow the same routine, except that they have to increase their calorie intake above the TDEE.

Remember, if you don't count your calories, your results won't be quantitative and you'll have to rely on hit and trial, so I suggest you do count your calories. Most of the food we consume has label indicating both macro (Protein, Carbohydrates,Fiber and Fat) and micronutrient content (Vitamins,Minerals).

LEAN MASS CALCULATION

Now we all know how to calculate our BMR, but it is to be noted that before calculating the BMR we should know the value of our body fat. Basically our body fat percentage decides if we need to calculate our BMR by considering our total body weight or our lean body mass. Lean Body Mass is basically the fat free mass in our body. It's also not your muscle mass so kindly don't get confused between the two. Normally if your body's fat percentage is more than 20 (in case of men)/28 (in case of women), it is advised to consider the lean mass to calculate the BMR.

There is a very simple formula that is been used to calculate the lean mass i.e.:

Lean Mass=Total body weight-(Body fat% * Total Body Weight).

For example, if a person is weighing 100kgs and has body fat % of 40 then his lean mass would be 100-(0.40*100)=60kgs. So the above person should calculate the BMR by putting his lean mass i.e. 60kgs instead of total body weight i.e. 100kgs.

Now I'd be giving out my personal diet but what worked for me, might not necessarily be working for you.

You know the saying "give a man a fish, you feed him once, teach a man how to fish and you feed him for a lifetime". I am going to do the latter. Many people are going to hate me for this.

I will discuss the following diets. Ratios for the macronutrients (carbs, protein, fat) are mentioned in the same order. Remember, these ratios aren't the biggest factor in determining your gain or loss of fat. What matters is your overall intake and overall expenditure and the difference is what stays or goes out of your body. However, these ratios and different diets help you follow a diet well, and has other aspects to it:

LOW CARB DIET (25:35:40)

This would be required to trim excess body fat, while making slow lean gains. It is effective, however takes a lot of time to show results (ideal for anyone who's new)

ZONE DIET (40:30:30)

This is the diet that has higher amounts of carbohydrates. This is ideal for the ones who absolutely love carbohydrates. This is also perfect for the people who have high tolerance towards carbohydrates which is commonly seen among the people with high muscle mass.

DEPLETION DIET (DYNAMIC)

To reduce body fat % dramatically and bring definition to your muscles in very short period (not for people with body fat above 10 %). This diet focuses mainly towards glycogen depletion and also reduces the subcutaneous water retension to a certain degree.

KETOGENIC DIET (5:35:60)

A ketogenic diet will also target your body fat levels and like the depletion diet, it will also reduce your water retention to a large extent. It engages your body in producing more ketones (will discuss in the diet sections) hence the name, Keto Diet. It is an ideal diet to start with if your goal is fat loss but would be sub-optimal for muscle gain.

I will also cover the carb loading. In brief however, since it is a very complex subject and a lot of research is still going on about it.

WARNING: Depletion diet requires immense knowledge and understanding about body composition and should only be attempted if you're an advanced level athlete and are below 10% body fat it can screw up your metabolism if done wrong, not to mention causing muscle loss and hormonal imbalance.

Before you start planning your diet, you have to calculate your BMR as mentioned before. Figure out how many calories you're going to consume to reach your target goal and then based on the diet, you have to divide your macronutrients into ratios.

REMEMBER, the BMR we calculated above only provides a baseline, many people have the metabolic rate above it or under it and therefore BMR should not be considered a universal indicator of one's metabolic rate.

LOW CARB DIET

Since we're looking to get shredded by low carb diet, our **Fat:carbs:protein Ratio** should be low in carbs and balanced protein and fats depending on the rest of our intake. **A 40:25:35 F:C:P** ratio is decent for this in most cases. of course there will be slight variation, but that is fine. It's just to give you an idea and stress on the fact that your carb intake will be the lower while fat intake will be the highest (keeping protein constant).

How does it helps? Fats help in satiety. And this diet will help you to stay satiated, with enough fiber of course. Also, it's good for anyone who's insulin resistant or diabetic (more on this later. do not experiment on your own if you are diabetic. Suggested an expert to handle such cases)

To help you understand more efficiently, let me give you an example

I am 28-year-old and 5'10" weighing 75kg, after calculating my BMR (say 2000) I calculate my daily calorie need using the Harris Benedict equation (mentioned above) and my calorie intake comes to about 2300 calories a day considering I do light exercise (just an example).

Now to start losing weight (fat, not muscles) I will design my diet in such a way that I will have a macro ratio of 20:45:30 in a calorie deficit mode. How many calories you need to reduce? It's up to you. However, the body does not like dramatic changes and it retaliates in a dramatic manner, leading to loose skin, water retention etc. (will address these problems in later part). It's better to lose weight gradually than dramatically. So I'd suggest a cut of 200-300 calories in first couple of weeks to start noticing change. And then further down by 400-500 in subsequent weeks to start fat loss and turn the body into a fat burning machine. You should never reduce more than 1000 calories, as it would most probably slow down your metabolism.

Protein has 4, Carb has 4 and Fat has 9 calories per gram.

So if I were to receive 2000 cals in a day, I will use the macro ratio of 40:25:35 to calculate my macro in grams.125 gm carbs, 175 gm protein and 89 gm of fat.

Now it is tough to find food which has only protein or carb or fat alone. Most of the foods have a mix of all. In this case you can look at the labels or use google and a little bit of brain to find out what combination will give you the above ratio.

MY PERSONAL DIET

So by now you must have understood that everyone owns a different car and I have my very own car. In this section, I'll tell you about how I fuel and maintain my car. Note that your car is different, so do not apply these to yourself.

However, here you go!

I try to keep things simple. The taste doesn't really matter to me as long as I am getting the desired results. Now some people won't be able to do that. I urge people to start a diet which they can sustain in the long run rather than copying from others for a short period only to eventually give up after getting frustrated.

Here's what I mostly eat:

I use eggs as my staple for protein, brown rice and oats for carbs, and nuts and flaxseeds for fats.

Keep the staple the same and you have the flexibility to play ground. For example, if I have to reduce my caloric intake, then instead of eating 100 gram brown rice, I'll eat 50gm, same for protein and fat. Monotony is a part of the deal, but don't forget – you cannot achieve what you desire for sitting in your comfort zone – You have to go walk the hard path!

And from my personal experience, it gets easier with time. Setting a goal of course is very important.

FOOD	CALORIE	PROTEIN,CARBS,FAT
AROUND 10 AM 1 Scoop Protein shake	121 cals	25 gm protein 3 gm carbs 1gm fat
AROUND 2PM 5 Whole eggs 1 Bowl Spinach 150 gm Mct Oil 1 Tbspn Fat free curd 100 gm	350+80+130+40 =600 cals	30 gm protein, 15 gm carbs, 45 gm fat
AROUND 6 PM		
AROUND 8 PM POST WORKOUT 2 Scoops Protein	242 cals	50 gm protein, 6gm carbs, 2gm fat
AROUND 9 PM 1 Bowl spinach 150 gm Mct oil 1 Tbspn Fat free curd 100 gm Brown rice 30 gms	80+130+40+150 cals =400 cals	Around 45 gms carbs, 20 gm fat, 5 gm protein.

AAROUND 10.30 PM 200 gms Boiled Chicken (breast) 6 Scrambled Eggs	220+102 =322 cals	60 gm protein, 5gm fat
1 AM Sleep		
TOTAL	**1685 cals**	**170gms protein,69 gms carbs,73 gm fat**

Alright, so this is my diet for the entire day and you can see that the above diet is not really perfect and is short of 2000 cals – This is to give you an idea. As I mentioned earlier, the aim here is to teach you how to catch the fish instead of feeding it to you. I'm sure you can now design a diet plan for yourself.

If you are curious about the high amount of green vegetables in the diet, here's the reason: First, they are very less in carbs/calories and give you a feeling of fullness, also known as satiety. So if you are eating in a deficit, fiber helps you stay full even at lower calories. And second, they provide you high amount of dietary fiber which is required for proper digestion of your protein. So please do not ignore fiber in your diet or it might lead to constipation or dehydration.

You can use the following table to choose your staples.

PROTEIN	CARBS	FATS	FIBER
Chicken	Green vegetables	Paneer	Vegetables
Eggs	Fruits	Yogurt	Sprouts
Fish	Rice	Cheese	Fruits
Whey protein	Legumes	Olive oil	
Tofu	Sprouts	Flaxseed	
White mushrooms	Banana	Fish oil	

Paneer/cheese	Wheat	Nuts	
Soy beans/ chunks	Quinoa	Coconut	

This limited list is only for your reference (in no particular order). There are several others you can choose from

ZONE DIET

Simply change the macro ratio in the above diet to 40:30:30 and it becomes Zone diet for lean muscle gains if you stay on a small surplus. However, if you keep total calories on a deficit, it will help you drop your body weight. You can introduce more carbs like oats, brown rice, sweet potato etc. It is always a good idea to consume carbs around the workout. What really matters

DEPLETION DIET

WARNING: Following a depletion diet without proper know-how can lead to severe consequences. You've been warned. Depletion diet is no child's play!

You will need iron will and a rock solid determination to complete two weeks of this diet. I would not suggest extending it beyond that period for multiple reasons including but not limited to hormonal damage, poor metabolism, and regaining weight. So if you do it, do it 100% right or do not do it at all.

It's called a Depletion Diet because you will deplete your body of carbohydrates and sugars, which will leave you with fat as the only available option in the body compelling it to make the "Switch" thereby allowing body to use fat as its primary fuel (of course, coupled with the right resistance training and proper protein intake)

Once again, I am not going to give you a magic formula. The idea here is to teach you, to help you understand how things work so that you can design your own diet. Now let's set a few things straight.

Your body including your muscle tissues is 70% water!

Your muscles are not as big as you think they are. They appear big at any point of time as holding a lot of glycogen and water in them. Generally, 100 gm of your lean muscle tissue will hold up to 2 gm of glycogen, and each of this 2gm of glycogen will further associate itself with around 3 grams of water.

So if a person has 30 kg of lean muscle tissue, i.e. 30,000gm of muscle tissue, the muscles will store up to 600gm of glycogen which will further store 600*3=1800gm of water. That's 1.8kg of water.

People who start with depletion diet often get confused when they see their weight dropping initially. It is this water glycogen weight that shows a massive drop initially. Even though there is no fat loss, you can lose up to 2 to 5kg of your bodyweight at the beginning of the diet depending on your lean muscle tissue and water storage capacity.

Feeling a bit disappointed? You shouldn't be! It is actually not a bad thing. If you are into a body building contest preparation, you will realize how this water and glycogen manipulation can make you stand out in the crowd (Has to do with bodybuilding. Others can ignore).

Well, let's get deeper.

So now you know that proper fat loss is not really an easy game and to start seeing any results, you will have to get your basics right. And that my friends, is the main idea behind any diet, be it Atkins diet, or low carb diet.

One way of doing that would be to gradually reduce the caloric intake. But returning to depletion diet, the goal would be to gradually reduce the carb intake every week or few days, so that eventually our intake is less than 20gm per day, and simultaneously, we'll be supplementing with enough protein to make sure muscle loss is minimum. And don't worry if your muscles appear flat, it's because your muscles are getting rid of the excess glycogen and water. They will fill out once you're back to your normal routine.

Also, the initial few days of carb depletion will be very challenging as your body will struggle to adjust with lower energy supplies. Remember at this point it will be reluctant to use fat as energy source. However once your glycogen levels are completely depleted, you will experience what is called "the switch" i.e. your body will start using fat and you will feel tremendous surge in your energy levels. This should happen typically during the second week. The key is to keep pushing through the first week.

The following is a sample depletion diet which I use. This is what I personally use, if you compare this with my normal diet (earlier chapters), you will notice that I have eliminated all source of carbs here except spinach (since we need dietary fiber at all times and the carb content in vegetables can be ignored).

I agree that this is neither an ideal diet, nor is it properly balanced. But then, I'm sharing it only to give you a rough idea. Now that you know the concept I am sure you can come up with a diet which looks perfect for you. You can even add other vegetables and protein sources in it.

FOOD	NOTE
AROUND 10 AM 1 Scoop Protein shake 1 tbsp Flaxseed 4 Egg white omelette	During the first week you can have brown rice as a measure of your carbs and you can gradually keep reducing it. E.g. 100gm, then 80, then 60 and so on and during the conditioning week, no brown rice.
AROUND 2 PM 8 EGG White scramble 1 bowl Spinach 200gm	
AROUND 6PM 4 Egg Whites	
AROUND 8PM POSTWORKOUT 2 Scoops Protein	
AROUND 10 PM 8 Scrambled Eggs 1 Bowl Spinach 200gm	
12 Am 1 scoop Protein (depends)	
1 AM	
Sleep	

Please note that you will have to drink more water than usual. Since your muscles will lose glycogen and consequently water, you will continuously need to drink water to replenish and keep them hydrated.

Let's move on to another very important diet.

THE KETOGENIC DIET

This has been a real hype in recent years. It has been treated as a God-sent magical diet. While it works great, trust me, it's no more superior to any other structured diet, considering only fat loss as the result, if you keep the basic variables the same, that is, your intake and your expenditure in terms of energy, your total protein intake and your training.

Let's get down to the basics.

Ketogenic diet or Keto is basically a diet where you will have absolutely minimum carbs say 20-30gms max. This will force the body to utilize fat as a primary source of fuel thereby aiding fat loss. Remember the car and the fuel example? There are different variations of Keto. One that is worth noting is the Atkin's version. In this version of Keto, you basically eat fat to burn fat. This is particularly good for people who face adherence issues when on a diet with carbs as keto forces you to stay strict to be in ketosis, a state where your body uses ketones and fatty acids as a source of fuel instead of glucose(although your brain always needs a supply of glucose to function. We'll talk about that later). Let's discuss the Atkins version of Keto along with a sample diet plan.

For Atkin's I suggest you use the 5:35:60 macro ratio i.e. 5 portions of Carbs, 35 portions of Protein and 60 portions of Fat.

Now for example, my BMR is around 1500 and my TDEE (total daily energy expenditure is 2000) so my macro breakdown for Keto will be:

25gms of Carbs, 200gms of Protein, and 122gms of Fat

Now we will build a sample diet around this. Like I've mentioned earlier, I like to keep things simple and hence I use food that I use daily and is easily available.

For **Atkins,** following are the **BEST CHOICES** for me

- Paneer (*per 100gm-Fat 20gm, Protein-20gm, Carb 1.5gm*)
- Amul Cheese (*1 slice-Fat 5gm,-Protein 4gm, Carbs-negligible*)
- Extra Virgin Coconut Oil (*per 100gm—Fat 86gm*)

- Flaxseed (*per 100gm-Fat 42gm,-Protein 18gm, Carbs 29gm*)
- Spinach (*or any other dark green vegetables for fiber*)

A sample diet would look something like this:

FOOD	NOTE
AROUND 8 AM Breakfast 50gm Paneer 1 Cheese Slice 4 Egg Whites	Paneer (per100gm fat20gm, protein-20gm, carb 1.5gm)
AROUND 11 AM 50gm Paneer 1 Cheese Slice	Amul cheese (1 slice-fat 5gm,-Protein 4gm, Carbs-negligible)
1 PM LUNCH 100 gm Paneer 1 bowl of spinach or any of your favourite vegetable	Spinach (or any other dark green vegetables for fibre)
Snacks, Paneer Cubes sauted in Extra Virgin Coconut Oil	Extra virgin coconut oil(100gm—fat86gm)
9PM DINNER 100gm Paneer 1 bowl of spinach or any of your favourite vegetable	

This was just an approximated version and the diet will vary for every individual. Let me remind you again that this information is to help you understand how to make a customized diet plan and not to give you a readymade plan.

Ketosis within your body will start typically 2-3 days after you start this diet and you will start seeing quick results soon. You may get a urine test done to see if your body is producing more ketones than usual, or you can simply test it with urine analysis sticks.

Most important thing is that you must, I am stressing on it again, keep off carbs completely. Carbs can completely reverse the effect of this diet.

Also if you lose 1-2kgs in initial 2-3 days, don't start jumping! Like I mentioned, it would be your water weight associated with the glycogen that will be depleted. Although, you can lose up to 4-5 kgs in 4 weeks of this diet (varies for every individual again)

Please note – A lot of people recommend a refeed to be done every week. However, from my experience, I have noticed that the body gets smooth and retains a lot of water. It is good idea to stay on Keto for at least 4 weeks continuously before having carbs again in a refeed.

Also sometimes, people start consuming more protein thinking it will help. However, it doesn't really help that way since you may get thrown out of ketosis with higher intake of protein too. It would be wise to have a higher protein intake in the initial weeks until the body gets keto adapted. Once ketosis is achieved, the protein intake can be reduced to around 15-20% of the diet.

CKD AND CHEAT MEALS

Cheat Meal is that meal in your diet where you can have any food that you like and it can be absolutely anything from a full-fledged ice cream sundae to your favorite biryani. Anyone with a body fat percentage below 10% can have cheat meal after an induction period of approximately 4 weeks of following ketogenic diet strictly. This is done to boost your leptin levels, which is one of the most critical hormones for losing fat. If you are getting results and your weight loss has not stalled, then there is no need for a cheat meal and you can just keep playing with your calories. Just don't bring it down to the levels you started with.

Cyclic Ketogenic Diet also popularly known as **CKD** should be followed by people who have body fat levels below 8%, People up to 10% can also follow it but they should have a decent amount of muscle mass.

The main principle behind cyclic ketogenic diet is the depletion and super compensation of your glycogen stores like I explained earlier. It is very critical for your sarcoplasmic growth. Now, even CKD can be done only once you are keto induced. So it is advised to follow a strict ketogenic diet for a period of at least 3-4 weeks. This induction phase is very important and further determines the success of your CKD. Some people tend to jump directly on CKD without getting properly induced, which is nothing short of a disaster.

So here is the correct method of doing CKD:

You have to get keto induced for a period of 3-4 weeks (make sure you are around 8% bf), then you move to CKD. You stay on keto for a period of 5-6 days (depending on your muscle mass, sensitivity towards carbs and a lot of other factors.

A typical CKD cycle for a week would look like this

MONDAY-Keto

TUESDAY-Keto

WEDNESDAY-Keto

THURSDAY-Keto

FRIDAY-Keto

SATURDAY morning, you need to do a depletion without (high intensity, full body, high volume, high repeatation workout done to make sure your glycogen levels are completely depleted) after which you will start taking a combination of glucose + protein, every 2 hours for the next 8 hours along with some simple carbs. In the subsequent 16 hours, you can take solid meals like rice, chicken, pasta, oats and anything else you want. The amount of carbs that you need to take, depends on your lean body weight. The typical formula is to have around 6-8gm per kg of your lean body weight, so for a 70kg guy with 10% bf, that would come at around 500-600gms of carbs. However, this formula is highly flawed and can often lead to excess carbs. Instead, I'd suggest eating 50gm carbs every 2 hours in the next 16 hours and see how your body reacts.

On SUNDAY morning, you should look fuller, more defined and more muscular. If you are holding water, or you are looking flat, it means, either the carbs were too less or they were too many. So it takes a little trial and error to hit the right amount. Again, this you will have to figure out on your own with some practice and see what for you.

On Sunday you can either continue to load carbs, or if you have had too many on Saturday and are holding water, then do some cardio to burn off the excess calories and you can switch to keto or eat carbs at your maintenance calories.

Some people make use of the period and do cheats as well, which is fine since everything you eat is primarily used by your body to fill up your depleted glycogen stores. So sweets, ice creams, candies, cookies, biryani etc. are all allowed, however make sure your total fat intake on these 1-2 days is less than 15% of your maintenance calories.

Also, make sure you do your depletion workout with maximum intensity, as the only way to super compensate your glycogen levels is by making sure it is completely depleted in the first place.

PEAK WEEK AND CONTEST PREPARATION

This is just for your information.

Remember when I said that during initial period of carb depletion, your body only loses water weight? And how that it is not a bad thing. Now I'll explain how.

See once your muscles are depleted of glycogen and water, they have a tendency to store more glycogen. If during normal state your muscles stored 2gm of glycogen per 100gm of lean muscle tissue, after depletion it can store up to 4gm of glycogen and hence more water. Bodybuilders and athletes take advantage of this situation. Following a depletion diet, they start carb loading, which lets them appear fuller and huge on stage and all the carb will get used up to fill increased glycogen levels. Also a lot of subcutaneous (under the skin) water will be pulled into the muscles giving a dry and ripped look. However, this only works for people who are below a body fat % of 10 or less, as it won't make a difference if you have more fat mass.

Not all Carbs are the same
Not all Calories are the same

Agreed it's the calories at the end of the day that matters when it comes to weight loss or weight gain, but choosing to ignore the right source because you read some new research or an article by some of the leading names in the industry may actually not be beneficial for your ultimate goals. You will get result, will the results be optimal? Far from it actually

So people professing that eating Dal chawal, mixing carbs and fats,eating sweets is allowed because it is within their TDEE. Here's something might burst your bubble:

Not all calories are treated in the same way by the body, for eg. Both fructose and glucose yield 4 calories per gm, but they are very different when it comes to being metabolized by the body. Fats have a different metabolic pathway so do amino acids, and mind you all this is conditional, based on different circumstances, the usage in the body can change.

One such example is the ghrelin levels. Ghrelin is your hunger hormone. When it is up, it makes you feel hungry. Different foods have different effects on ghrelin levels, while foods containing fructose or glucose will trigger more ghrelin levels and will make you eat more compared to proteins or facts. This is one more reason why it is easy to stick to a low carb diet compared to a high carb diet at the same calories.

Different foods can impact your metabolism negatively or positively, be on ice-cream diet for 1600 calories for a few days and you'll see your metabolism will drop and even at 1600 calories you will find it difficult to lose weight. Try the same with a high protein or a high fat diet and you'll be losing weight pretty sharply. Same calories and different results, anyone doubting the results can try it on themselves if they dare

A gram of omega-3 fatty acid will provide the same amount of calories as a gram of omega-6 fatty acids, yet one is good while other is bad for health (read: high amount of omega-6 in our existing diets).

So you see a calorie is not just a calorie, and anyone who says that at the end of the day that calories are calories and source dosen't matter does not know that they are talking about.

Sources of the calories matter! Be wise, while picking the sources.

REVERSE DIETING

You hit a wall!

The single most relevant factor that is responsible for a 'no-more' fat loss zone or fat loss plateau is the down regulation/slowdown of your metabolism. This is because as you cut down calories, no matter how small the deficit be, metabolism will start to come down. Simply because the body will try to preserve energy for survival. In the process our body will reduce the production of metabolism friendly hormones like thyroid, free testosterone and leptin to maintain energy balance. Not just that, but your body will downregulate a lot of its operations.

Reverse Dieting protocol:

Now you might claim that decreasing calories result in weight loss, so adding up calories will result gain. This is where maintenance calories have to be kept in mind while reverse dieting specifically for weight loss. A slight increase in weight while reverse dieting dose not necessarily mean that you are adding fat. That will not happen unless you go beyond your maintenance

Calories or over look macro distribution. This slight increase in weight will be intra cellular water retention or gain in muscle glycogen. For example, if u are on a calorie deficit diet for weight loss, you start off by preparing a diet chart with calories equal to your BMR = 1600 calories and you are following a low carb diet so you would start with calculating your macros for 1600 calories i.e. 25:45:30 – C/P/F. this would come up to 80gms carbs, 160gms proteins and 71gms fat. Now after following a chart with the mentioned macros for a week, you should increase the calories by 100-150 gms (depends upon the week's result) so for the next week you will have to modify your diet chart and make a new chart for 1600 + 100 = 1700 calories, similarly the macros would change to 85gms carbs, 170gms proteins and 75gms fat. Every week we keep increasing the calories by 100-150 based on the improvement and keep repeating the procedure till our fat loss stalls. The stage at which this happens, this stalling, this stage indicates that the person has reached his/her maintenance calories and thus they should ideally go back to their BMR value and repeat the whole thing again.

DIETING ROAD MAP

Most of the people after reading this would like to start dieting immediately, without any clue as to what they will do once it's all over. Shall they repeat the dieting or go back to their old habits. That is what I will cover in this section.

DIETING STRATEGY – Everyone wants to get muscles, but u have to decide for yourself. Do you want to look like a freak show or aesthetically built? If the answer is latter, then you should follow this guideline

- If you can see your abs, you can start by adding around 150-200kcals to your maintenance calorie with low carb diet initially for 4 weeks and then continue on zone diet for as long as you want.
- If can't see your abs but are already fit, then switch to low carb till you are shredded enough and then stick to zone diet for as long as you want. Whichever diet you choose for dropping your fats or for gaining muscles, you need to maintain a calorie deficit or a calorie surplus respectively.

  Do not keep reducing the calories – most people, if they don't get results, keep on reducing calories further and further, which is not good. What you are actually doing is you are harming your metabolism. This is true for most people who tend to lose weight by doing a starvation or crash diet. And they gain the weight back again very soon. Read this article on how you get fat eventually by eating lesser and lesser.

  If you do the above mentioned diets correctly, you will see that your metabolism will only get better, you may even keep losing weight despite higher calorie intake however, you should be regularly lifting heavy weights as well. Your training and work out should be on point. Not only during the dieting down phase, but always.

REMEMBER, the more muscles you have, the more fat body will burn, even while resting. So focus on building muscles. This is applicable to both genders nothing like women should not! However, this is just one of the many strategies that can be used to achieve the desired body composition. You are free to choose what works best for you.

TRAINING

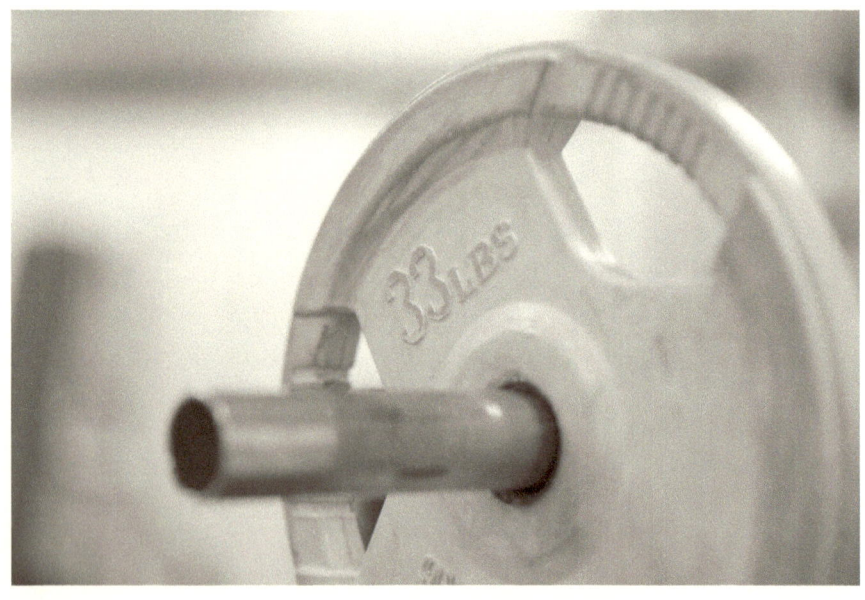

TRAINING FOR THE "MEN"

If I were to get a dollar every time someone asked whether they should go for heavy weight, less rep or light weight, more repeatations I'd probably be a millionaire.

There are lot of factors that matter when it comes to building muscles or losing fat, ranging from body type to genetic and what not. Different type of sports would require you to have different bodies, however since we're into building muscles and losing fat, I'll only discuss training which will be relevant to that.

Starting with body type, we have three major classification:

1. ECTOMORPH
   An ectomorph is the typical skinny guy. Ectomorphs have a light build with small joints and lean muscle. Usually ectomorphs have long time limbs with stringy muscles. Shoulders tend to be thin with little width.

2. MESOMORPH
   A mesomorph has a large bone structure, large muscles and a naturally athletic physique. Mesomorphs are the best body type for bodybuilding. They find it quite easy to gain and lose weight. They are naturally strong which makes for the perfect platform to build muscle.

3. ENDOMORPH
   The endomorph body type is solid and generally soft. Endomorphs gain fat very easily. Endomorphs are usually of a shorter build with thick arms and legs. Muscles are strong, especially the upper legs. Endomorphs find they are naturally strong in leg exercises like the squat.

   Now don't be disheartened if you are an ectomorph or endomorph.

   Since your primary goal is to build (or maintain) muscles, you need to understand them first.
   Your muscles are not all the same size, and may require different types of stimulus to get stronger and developed. You cannot keep doing squats and expect to get a good chest-I know that is obvious and it is not what I am trying to say, what I mean to say is that the weight, the repetitions,

the intensity and the form, all these are the factors that play an important part in giving the proper stimulus to any muscle group. So if you were going to ask should I lift heavy weight and do less reps or lift lightweight and do more reps, read what I just said again. There is no single answer and no one size fits all here. Different athletes in the history of bodybuilding have showed and proved that you can build a great body by following different methods.

MUSCLE FIBER TYPES

Though muscles are muscles, their composition can vary. It can have different proportions of two different kinds of muscle fibers-slow twitch and fast twitch.

So your body has bundles of muscle fibers, and these bundles have varying proportions of these two types of fibers.

1. SLOW TWITCH
   These are also known as type 1 or red muscle fibers. They are responsible for long-duration, low intensity activity such as walking or any other aerobic activity.

2. FAST TWITCH
   These are known as Type 2 or white muscle fibers (divided further into A and B) They are responsible for short-duration, high intensity activity. **TYPE 2B** fibers are built for explosive, very short-duration activity such as Olympic lifts. **TYPE 2A** fibers are designed for short-to moderate duration, moderate-to-high intensity work, as is seen in most weight training activities.

By looking at elite athletes in different sports, you can see extreme examples of each make-up of muscle fiber. At the slow twitch end is the endurance athlete, such as the marathon runner.

These athletes can have up to 80% or more of slow twitch muscle fibers in their bodies, making them extremely efficient over long distances. At the fast twitch end is the sprinter. World-class sprinters can have up to 80% or more of fast twitch muscle fibers in their body, making them extremely fast, strong and powerful but with limited endurance.

HOW TO TRAIN YOUR MUSCLE FIBER TYPE?

When you're training with weights, your goal is to work as many muscle fibers as possible. Targeting more muscle fibers means greater gains in strength and muscle mass.

If your fibers in a particular muscle consist primarily of slow twitch fibers, in order to affect the greatest number of those muscle fibers, you'll need to train that muscle with higher reps, shorter rest periods and higher volume. This is because they take longer to fatigue, they recover quickly and they require more work to maximize growth.

Unfortunately, slow twitch muscle fibers are limited in their potential for growth so even if a muscle group is primarily slow twitch, you should definitely include some lower rep training to maximize the fast twitch fibers you've got in that muscle.

If you find you have a hard time gaining size in particular muscle, it could be because it has a predominance of slow twitch muscle fibers. Higher reps (e.g.12to15reps), higher volume (more sets) and shorter rest periods (30 seconds to a minute between sets) can help you to maximize those muscles.

This doesn't mean you should use light weight, though. You should still strive to use weights that are as heavy as possible that will cause you to reach failure in those higher rep ranges. If you don't use heavy weights, you won't give your muscles a reason to grow.

If your fibers in a particular muscle group consist primarily of fast twitch muscle fibers, you're one of the lucky ones. You'll have a much easier time building mass in that muscle-fast twitch muscle fibers have greater potential for size than slow twitch. The more fast twitch fibers you've got, the greater your quickest to develop.

To maximize your muscles with fast twitch fibers, you'll need to train with low to moderate reps (e.g.4 to 8 reps), rest period so far around 1 to 2 minutes and a moderate training volume (too much volume will compromise recovery).

If your muscles have a fairly even mix of fibers, you can evenly divide your training between focusing on the lower-rep, fast twitch fiber training and the higher-rep, and slow twitch fiber training. This will help you to develop all the fibers in your muscles, maximizing your ultimate development.

TIME UNDER TENSION OR T.U.T

Although you have read the above article, science claims that irrespective of the weights, your muscles develop when they are put under tension for certain duration which crosses your muscles threshold. For eg. You can lift a 20 kg dumbbell and do 5-8 reps or you can hold a kg dumbbell facing upwards and hold it for a minute. So which one is difficult? Which one will give you more benefit? The light weight or the heavy? As both the weights will put your bicep muscle under immense tension for a certain duration. Food for thought! Next time someone asks you in the gym to lift the heaviest possible weight, ask them to hold the smallest possible weight against gravity for certain duration.

Follow these tips for optimum results:

- Use drop sets and super sets as tools for more volume in workout. Volume is all that matters.
- Do more inclined chest press as it will build your overall chest.
- Like I said, volume is the key. Instead of doing chest press. This will minimize the load on your shoulders and maximize the load on your chest.
- Follow a 1:3 approach, 1 second to pick the weight up and 3 seconds to bring it down slowly.
- Do it slow and do it in proper form
- Use dumbbells wherever possible instead of barbells. It will isolate each side.
- Weighted pull-ups is one of the best exercises: do it everyday. Even if you are able to do one, do it with strict form.
- With back, its mostly pull, so you have to lift heavy enough weights.
- Try to avoid exercises which hurt your neck, Lat pulldown behind neck is a big no-no.
- Use compound movements.
- Focus on your negatives and try to hold the weight, Mind-muscle Connection.
- Do heavy lifting, but not ego lifting.
- Don't overlook calves and hamstrings. You're going to get lot of negativity if you don't focus on them, especially the calves.

Also since cardio is a big thing among gym goers, let's go ahead and cover that too.

CARDIO

Cardiovascular exercises or cardio are basically any exercises that can raise your heart rate. They are beneficial for your overall cardiovascular health I.e. your heart and your respiratory system. Cycling, running on treadmill, or cross-fit trainer are a few examples of cardio. Cardio can be done once or multiple times throughout the week. However, doing cardio for weight loss is not a suitable option for multiple reasons. Rather change your diet.

Research has shown doing regular cardio can significantly improve your cardiovascular health: however, it should not be used for dropping inches off your body. From my personal experience, weight training is the best way to do it.

HIIT Vs Steady State Cardio.

HIIT or high intensity interval training is basically a training split in which your resting periods are smaller. An example would be to run on treadmill for 2 minutes at 15kmph and then taking a gap of 1 minute and then running again. HIIT assist in gaining muscles and is shown to increase your metabolism over a 24-hour period. HIIT is fueled by both glycogen and fat and will not target fat immediately. Some researchers have proved however that doing HIIT will help you reduce more overall calories in shorter amount of time than steady state cardio.

My Opinion?

HIIT is a real monster and does what it claims. However, it is pretty exhaustive!

Steady state cardio – is cardio done in 70-75% of your maximum heart rate range. It taps your fat for energy and is very effective for dropping the last few pounds before a show. You can still do it for overall good cardiovascular health but do not expect magic!

Use cardio for improving your cardiovascular health. You are not going to build any muscle while on cardio and remember, the more muscles you have, the more fat you burn even while you're resting so it's your call to make.

If you're looking for a personal training regimen, I'd suggest downloading Bodyspace app, It is a free app from bodybuilding.com and has more than 40000 training programs.

MY BEST EXCUSE FOR AVOIDING CARDIO FOR FATLOSS!

Like everyone, even a normal man before paying his annual membership fees of the gym he wanted to join, checked out their equipment for cardio: there were 8 treadmills, 6 bicycles and 6 cross trainers (or elliptical, whatever). He felt like he had found the perfect gym. Paid his annual fees and from the next day itself, he started with 40 minutes of cardio utilizing all three of the different equipment for cardio and after that proceeded for 45 minutes more of weight training, because "big biceps are more important". A month passed, and he had lost around 3kgs and he was so relieved. Moreover, those figures on the equipment that displayed "calories burnt" felt like they were the right estimates and they may even have been right. But when he looked at himself in the mirror, there were no 'cuts' or 'blown up biceps'. It felt like the obsess aunty in the cardio room (who used the bicycle while talking on the phone) had the same progress as he had.

Diet was the obvious answer to all queries. So let me emphasize more on what cardio does and does not do, what can be its substitute for improving your cardiovascular health and most importantly, to burn your fats.

WHY ISN'T CARDIO THE FIRST OPTION FOR FAT LOSS?

The basic idea behind doing cardio for losing fats for an average person is, you burn more calories and hence your total caloric expenditure is more than your caloric intake and this isn't wrong by any means. But do we know from where our body is making arrangements for these calories needed? Yeah, some fats are burned here, but after a short while your body starts breaking muscles for converting them into glucose which will be used as energy by the body. There was a study done where subjects were examined for 4 months where one group did low intensity cardio while the other did high intensity cardio for 4 months and it was concluded that there was a significant loss of muscle mass in the subjects that did the low intensity cardio whereas, surprisingly, there was a slight increase in the muscle mass in the subjects doing high intensity interval cardio.

Now this muscle loss will further bring down your metabolism because muscles eat up energy and since you are burning your muscles, less energy will be expended.

Why does this happen? Because the cortisol levels increase in your body when you perform low intensity cardio. Cortisol is a stress hormone which mainly causes muscle breakdown when cardio is done in isolation without any resistance training.

- *Low intensity cardio is where you jog at a moderate to low speeds for a prolonged duration*
- *High intensity cardio is where you run at your highest speed and it becomes interval cardio when you add periodic intervals in between.*

WHAT IS THE ALTERNATIVE TO CARDIO THEN, you ask?

Here are two options before you:

- **Strength training and low intensity steady state cardio:**

Strength training and cardio both can help. ST helps in retaining muscle or even better, building muscle. Cardio will help in additional fat loss apart from helping with improving the cardiovascular health.

- **Strength training and high intensity interval training:**

This needs a detailed explanation. Let us begin.

Now, when you're doing low intensity cardio, you start breathing faster because you need more energy and your body derives this energy by sending oxygen to your muscles causing the muscles to break down into glucose and then providing you with energy. But when you're doing HIIT or strength training, your body needs the energy faster. It simply cannot wait for the oxygen anymore. Here the body causes the increase in the levels of lactate. The glucose is broken down into pyruvate which is converted into lactate and this is sent to the liver to be again converted into glucose to be used as energy.

[Glucose>pyruvate>lactate>glucose=energy]

Glucose is again used here like it was used in LISS so how are we sparing the muscles here? The thing is, unlike in the former, here not only your cortisol levels be elevated but even your growth Hormone and Testosterone levels go up. And in this environment, your body will burn fat and not the muscles!

One more advantage in HIIT is that, as the lactate levels go up, the capacity of your muscles to go on for some more time comes down. There is an upper limit for the presence of lactate too. In HIIT, we go above that limit when we are running at the highest pace. But even as we stop or start walking suddenly, the brain is under the impression that the lactate levels are over the top and so effect to this, the ability of our muscles to go on comes down. Now this prevents us from overtraining too which otherwise would cause breakdown of the muscles.

The environment in your body is different in LISS and HIIT. For example. Let's relate this action of 'running' to rain. When it rains in a drought prone area like Rajasthan, it's a boon, whereas if it rains in places where floods are common like Assam, it's not that great, is it? Exactly the same is the case here. When you 'run', cortisol levels go up, but when it's done HIIT style, it's like in Rajasthan: the situation is ideal as testosterone and growth hormone levels are hugh too resulting in just the fat loss. It's not the same in LISS. That's like in ASSAM, where you will save water in the dam and similarly here you will burn fats surely, but there will be bigger destruction like loss if some muscle mass.

Benefit of HIIT:

In HIIT you run at your highest speed for 30-45 seconds (this may vary with person to person) and then stop or walk for a minute or so and repeat. You cannot do this for half as long as you did low intensity cardio. This is still just an example. You can do HIIT in quite a lot of different ways.

SUPPLEMENTATION

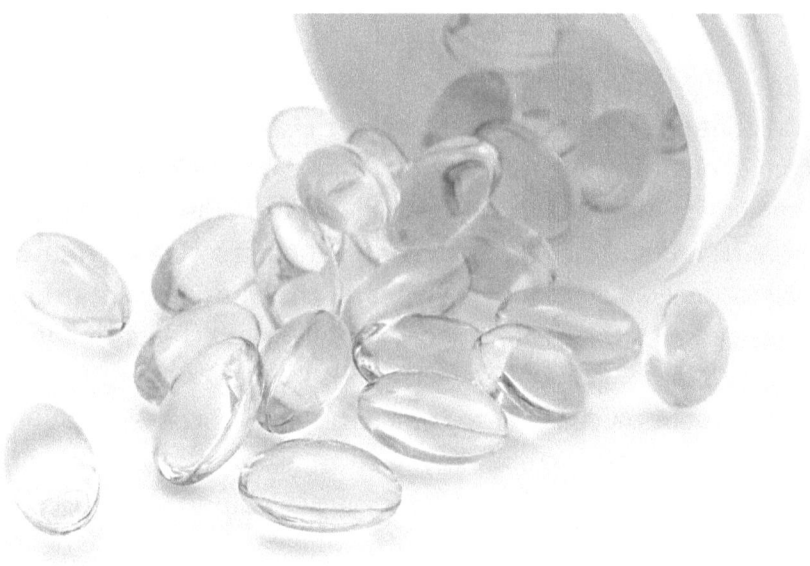

There are N numbers of supplements available in the market these days, be it L-Carnitine, HMB,CLA,NO products and so on and if you start buying them all, you'll probably have no money left in your pocket. See these products work, they have years of solid research backing up their claims, but they are pretty costly and for few unaffordable. Here let's see the most basic and most essential supplements.

PROTEIN

Not going to discuss this! You need this no matter how good your diet is, don't fall for expensive isolates though, blends are good too, 1.6-1.8gm per kg of lean body weight is required amount.

CREATINE

It gives you more energy to lift!

Quite literally!

When lifting heavy weights, your body primarily uses ATP and CP (Creatine phosphate) stores, however these are very limited and you cannot push any further until body makes more ATP from glycogen again. Also most of this ATP actually exists in the body in the form of ADP (adenosine di-phosphate). When creatine monohydrate is introduced in the body. It binds to the phosphorous inside the body and exists as creatine phosphate. Now this creatine phosphate during heavy workouts gives its phosphate to ADP to form ATP, this happens much faster than glycogen to ATP conversion thereby there's a notable increase in your strength. Creatine is one of the most well researched supplements available in the market and should be used by anyone who lifts weight.

Now there's a common myth that creatine retains water. So let's address that. First of all, what do you mean by water retention? The water is stored in your muscle cells as well as outside of your muscle cells under the skin.

This extracellular water stored under the skin is called Water Retention. It's a defense mechanism employed by the body to keep you hydrated all the time. Now creatine draws water directly into the muscles and not into the extracellular skin, which is a good thing. There is a lot of confusion about this. Most of the time, these people stop drinking water all together and stop consuming sodium as well. Now sodium is one major electrolyte that helps in regulation of water in the body. So when body detects low levels of sodium and water, the hormone aldosterone is triggered, which further as a part of body's defense mechanism tries to hang onto water, thereby causing water retention intracellular as well as extracellular. And people thought it was due to creatine.

BCAA

You don't really need it if you have enough protein intake which have complete amino acid profile. BCAA or branched chain amino acids are basically essential amino acids which are synthesized in the body, namely leucine, isoleucine and valine along with many other amino acids. However, what makes these BCAA's more important is the role that play. These amino acids are being used by the body for energy when you're lifting heavy weights. And if body starts making these amino acids it will not manufacture other amino acids at the same speed. And we know that all the amino acids are required for building proteins which are nothing but chains of amino acids. So it is always a good idea to supplement these essential amino acids, thereby giving body enough time to make all other amino acids, further leading to more muscle protein synthesis. However, if your protein intake for your body is sufficient, then you do not need to supplement with BCAA.

ZMA

ZMA or Zinc Magnesium Aspartate is a mineral supplement that is a combination of Zinc Monomethionine Aspartate, Magnesium Aspartate and Vitamin B6. The reason ZMA has become popular amongst athletes and people who do resistance training is because it supplements mainly with zinc and magnesium which is studied to be deficient in people who train.

Zinc has been proven to be vital for the activity of more than 100 enzymes. Zinc containing enzymes aid in macronutrient metabolism and cell replication, which as we know are key biochemical functions that corresponds to recovery and growth. Zinc has shown to have positive effects on anabolic hormone profile, particularly testosterone. It increases free serum testosterone levels which is particularly important in older men as their testosterone levels start to decline with age.

MICRONUTRIENTS

Your Multivitamin/multimineral tabs. They come cheap, and it's a good idea to take them.

You may not realize this but if your diet doesn't have chromium in it, you will suffer poor metabolism. How?

Let me explain, even though chromium is required in micrograms, it is an essential cofactor for proper functioning of your hormone insulin. And you know how important insulin is. This is just one example showing how important these micronutrients in your body can be. There are a total of more than 6 such vitamins and minerals that are required for optimum health by your body everyday. Unfortunately, there is no single food that will provide you the full spectrum, hence supplementation becomes all the more essential. Multivitamins and minerals tabs can do that for you.

Having a balanced diet can take care of most of the micronutrients however supplementation of the following is always beneficial and is even recommended:

Vitamin C, and for vegetarians-Vitamin-B (Thiamin, riboflavin, niacin, and so on).

Don't forget fish oil capsules or flaxseed oil for omega-3 and omega-6 fatty acids. Remember they are required by your brain. Similarly, garlic is a very beneficial herb.

ZMA IMPORTANCE

It is not really necessary if you have ample intake of these minerals from your diet. But if not, you might want to consider its use. Lower levels of zinc and magnesium are either due to sweating while training where you lose a lot of minerals and electrolytes or due to poor diet.

ZMA improves sleep-studies show that people suffering from mild to moderate insomnia seem to improve with oral magnesium therapy. Long term sleep deprivation causes magnesium deficiency and improving the magnesium intake can help with sleep. ZMA improves REM (rapid eye movement) cycles of the sleep. The better your sleep, more you recover and assimilate nutrients.

HORMONES

This is vast subject and medical jargon but one needs to understand.

So what are hormones?

Hormones are special chemical messengers that pass messages between different parts of your body and control various important functions in your body. They co-ordinate complex processes like growth, fertility and metabolism. You have facial hair? Hormones. You have good muscles naturally? Hormones. You feel very energetic? Hormones. Your menstruation to your thyroid functions-hormones. You are diabetic? Well, hormones.

Let's look at a few important hormones.

1. **Insulin –**
   Insulin has always been propagated as the muscle building hormone and even as the fat storing hormone. Truth is, it does both and you don't need to fret much about it. It's a hormone that helps you stay stable, by keeping your blood glucose levels stable when it tends to rise due to incoming carb intake. It "opens up" the cells to take the incoming glucose in.

   Insulin is a hormone made by the pancreas that allows your body to use sugar (glucose) from carbohydrates in the food that you eat for energy or to store glucose for future use. Insulin helps keeps your blood sugar level from getting too high (hyperglycemia) or too low(hypoglycemia).

   The cells in your body need sugar for energy. However, sugar cannot go into most of your cells directly. After you eat food and your blood sugar level rises, cells in your pancreas (known as beta cells) are signaled to release insulin into your bloodstream. Insulin then attaches to and signals cells to absorb sugar from the bloodstream. Insulin is often described as a "key", which unlocks the cell to allow sugar to enter the cell and be used for energy.

2. **Glucagon –**
   We discussed how insulin helps keep the blood glucose level stable by helping the body take in the excess glucose. Glucagon does the exact opposite by helping the blood glucose remain stable by bringing in supply of glucose when blood glucose is low, by breaking down the stored glycogen in the liver. So insulin and glucagon are interlinked, and it's no surprise that both of them are produced in the pancreas itself.

3. **Testosterone –**
   Now testosterone is the primary male hormone which gives men their "male" characteristic, from voice to facial hair. It helps maintain proper health in men and also helps build muscles. Now testosterone is a male hormone, but it doesn't mean that women don't produce it. Even women produce it, but much lesser than men. Women are more sensitive to this hormone. A healthy testosterone level is important for you for proper muscle gain and fat loss. So make sure your micronutrients are on point and that you are not a hypocaloric diet for long. (Note – there is a difference between calorie deficit and hypocaloric. Hypocaloric diet here means severe deficit for a long time.) The best testosterone booster in nature is lifting heavy weights. If you lift weights, your testosterone production gets better, thereby aiding in muscle build up and strength gains (in women, "toning" is essentially muscle build up itself, along with fat loss. Lifting weights will help you do instead of aerobics)

4. **Estrogen –**
   Estrogen is the female counterpart of testosterone. It makes a woman, a woman. It is responsible for the development and regulation of the female reproductive system and secondary sex characteristics. Now there are several different types of estrogen too, but that is beyond the scope of this book for now. One thing to remember here is, it is a very important hormone for women. And lifting weights will NOT bring it down to affect your health. Another concern among men is about the increase of estrogen in their bodies due to soya consumption. That won't happen unless you eat 1 kilo raw soya everyday continuously for months at a stretch. So there's nothing to worry about.

5. **Leptin –**

   Leptin is a very important hormone in your body that's essential for fat loss. It is like your fuel indicator that signals your brain about the availability of food, and based on that your brain holds on to your body's fat stores or goes easy on them to release them for use. That's directly related to metabolic adaptation (how your body controls and varies your metabolism). This hormone goes down when you are on a caloric deficit for too long, and the effect is more if carbs are omitted from the diet. This is the reason why a refeed helps. A well-timed and well-placed refeed can help you lose more by raising your leptin levels after a short dieting phase.

6. **Ghrelin –**

   This hormone is also known as the hunger hormone. It signals your body to feed it more. This hormone goes up when are on a caloric deficit for long and are dieting up. That's why you feel hungry. So the next time you feel hungry, don't think that your body lacks energy or energy stores. It has a lot of fat stores that it can use. It's just the ghrelin in action.

7. **Cortisol –**

   In the fitness community, cortisol is seen as the villain. Truth is, it is neutral. Depends on how it functions and the scenario it functions in. It is a catabolic hormone that helps in the metabolism of fat, protein and carbohydrate – all three. So even your fat loss is dependent on cortisol. However, excess amounts of cortisol for extended time periods is bad as it can metabolise your muscle mass too. Cortisol is released in response to stress and low blood glucose concentration. Minimize your stress, be on a good diet and make sure you take your micronutrients. Get involved in activities that you like doing. Pursue a hobby, meditate. It will not just help you with your cortisol but also lead a good life. Health is not only in your body but also in your mind.

SPECIALLY FOR WOMEN

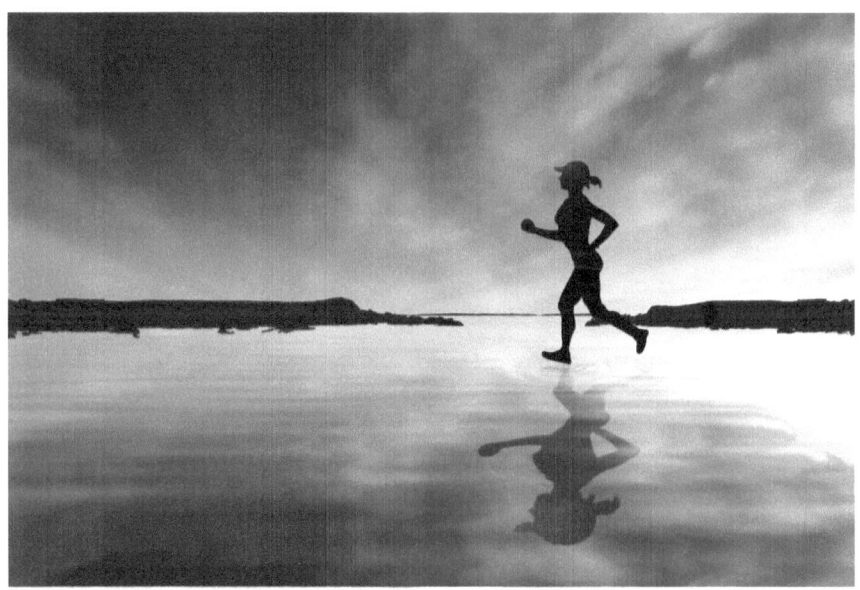

Youth and Beauty – it's always been assumed that the two go hand-in-hand. The sweet bird of youth stays for a brief summer but before long, it has flown away and its loss is lamented forever.

Humans value youth above all else. Society assumes that as youth passes, beauty fades away as well. Women, in particular, are judged quite harshly for being over a certain age. That's why more money has been spent on the vain search for the fountain of eternal youth than on anything else. While life expectancy has improved over time, it is still assumed that beyond a certain age, human health will inevitably decline.

But this need not be the case. There is tonnes of research that shows that the old assumption – advanced age equals decrepitude – can easily be proven wrong with a proper nutrition and training program.

Let's look at some important tips on staying fit and healthy over the age of 40:

- Weight Training

It's not a matter of debate anymore that women need to lift weights. Endless cardio and pink dumbbells may keep you thin but they won't make you fit.
Age-related Muscle Loss or Sarcopenia is a major problem for women over 50. However, the damage could start soon after 30 especially if one has an inactive lifestyle. Women who lead sedentary lives could lose as much as 3 to 5% muscle loss per decade which will only worsen with age.

Some form of Resistance Training is needed if women want to hold on to their curves and strength. Weight training is by far the best form of training. And no, women don't need to worry about looking like The Rock – your body simply doesn't produce the amount of testosterone needed to gain that much muscle.

If you can't or don't want to go to gym, you can still work up a sweat with Resistance Bands and Bodyweight Exercises right in the comfort of your homes.

What works: Lifting Heavy, Some Other Form Of Resistance Training.

What doesn't work: Endless Cardio, Light Weights, Bollywood Dance.

- **Protein**

Proteins have rightly been called the building blocks of our body. Without adequate amounts of this macronutrient (the others being Carbohydrates and Healthy Fats), the human body will break down and waste away.

There are far too many myths and horror stories about how too much protein can cause everything from weight gain to kidney failure. But how much is too much?

The Recommended Dietary Allowance (RDA) for protein is pretty low: just 0.8 grams of protein per kg of bodyweight. **Take a minute and calculate how much that means for *you.***

The RDA is the minimum amount of protein your body needs as below this level, your body faces imminent shutdown. If you're surprised to find that you're barely making the mark, trust me, you aren't alone.

If you're physically active, then your body needs more protein. Depending on the level of activity and intensity, you could need anywhere from 1 to 2 grams of protein per kg of bodyweight.

But will protein make you gain weight? Not if you eat at a caloric deficit or at maintenance. To know this, you need to take into account everything that you eat and drink, not just protein.

So don't believe the scaremongers – protein is an essential tool in your anti-aging arsenal!

- **Vitamin D**

Women often complain that they feel weak, no matter how rested they are. They're plagued with aches and pains and feel a general listlessness and lack of vigour. Their hair's falling out and they feel gloomy.

It isn't okay to feel this way and often, the culprit is low Vitamin D levels.

There are two forms of the "Sunshine Vitamin":

- Vitamin D2 or ergocalciferol – found in plant foods, supplements or fortified foods
- Vitamin D3 or cholecalciferol – found in animal foods, supplements/fortified foods and produced by our bodies when it comes into contact with sunlight

Vitamin D deficiencies are commoner than you'd think. Even though we live in a sub-tropical country, we spend most of our time indoors. Vegetarians are also at a greater risk of developing a deficiency on account of their dietary restrictions.

Long-term effects of a deficiency are increased risk of osteoporosis, cardiovascular diseases, auto-immune disease, certain forms of cancer, to name but a few.

The only definitive way to know if you're deficient is by taking a lab test. Do not self medicate; consult a physician or nutrition consultant who'd be able to guide you.

- **More Sleep, Less Stress**

In a world filled with distractions and brightly lit screens (TV/smartphones/iPads), how does one manage to get more than 5-6 hours of quality sleep a night?

Well, you better find a way if you want to remain healthy over 40. Late nights and early mornings may have been fine when you were younger but as you age, they start taking a toll on your health and appearance that even heavy make-up won't be able to hide.

You may workout, you may be eating right but if you're not getting adequate amounts of sleep, you're setting yourself up for illness.

Aim for 7-8 hours of quality restful sleep every night.

Other ways to get more sleep and reduce stress:

- Avoid watching TV or using your smartphone an hour before bedtime
- Keep your smartphone on silent and away from you when you go to bed. Turn off notifications so you're not disturbed while sleeping
- Avoid caffeine after 4 pm
- Make sure the bedroom is neither too cold nor too hot
- Meditate
- Keep a Daily Gratitude Journal. Every night before sleeping, write out 5 things that you are thankful for or 5 things that went well that day. People who follow this practice tend to feel less stressed out and get better sleep

Just because you're a woman over 40 does not mean your life is over and you should now spend your time in anticipation of meeting the Grim Reaper. By following a few easy steps and taking care of your health, the quality of your life will not only improve but may well be better than it was in your 20s.

APPENDIX

CALORIE-CHART 1

Item	Quantity	Caloric Value	Item	Quantity	Caloric Value
Breakfast			**Beverages**		
Egg Boiled	1	80	Tea, black, no sugar	1 cup	10
Egg Fried	1	110	Coffee, black, no sugar	1 cup	10
Egg Omelette	1	120	Tea with milk & sugar	1 cup	45
Bread slice with butter	1	90	Coffee, milk & sugar	1 cup	45
Chapati	1	60	Milk without sugar	1 cup	60
Puri	1	75	Milk with sugar	1 cup	75
Paratha	1	150	Horlicks, milk & sugar	1 cup	120
Subji	1 cup	150	Fresh fruit juice	1 cup	120
Idli	1	100	Aerated soft drinks	1 bottle	90
Dosa Plain	1	120	Beer	1 bottle	200
Dosa Masala	1	250	Soda	1 bottle	10
Sambhar	1 cup	150	Alcohol, neat	1 peg, small	75

Lunch/ Dinner			Miscellaneous		
Cooked rice, plain	1 cup	120	Jam	1 tsp	30
Cooked rice, fried	1 cup	150	Butter	1 tsp	50
Phulka	1	60	Ghee	1 tsp	50
Naan	1	150	Sugar	1 tsp	30
Dal	1 cup	150	Biscuit	1	30
Curd	1 cup	100	Fried nuts	1 cup	300
Curry, vegetable	1 cup	150	Puddings	1 cup	200
Curry, meat	1 cup	175	Ice-Cream	1 cup	200
Salad	1 cup	100	Milk shake	1 glass	200
Papad	1	45	Wafers	1 pkt	120
Cutlet	1	75	Samosa	1	100
Pickle	1 tsp	30	Bhel puri/ pani puri	1 helping	150
Soup, clear	1 cup	75	Kabab	1 plate	150
Soup, heavy	1 cup	150	Indian sweet/ mithai	1 pc	150
			Fruit	1 helping	75

CALORIE VALUE OF FOOD ITEMS
(Figures given in this chart are based on 100 gm portions)

Food	Calories	Protein (gms)	Fat (gms)	Carbohydrate (gms)	Water (gms)	Vitamins
Milk	65	2.3	4	5	87	A, B2, Niacin
Butter	740	–	82	–	15	A
Cream	210	2	21	3	72	A
Cheese	310	22	25	–	44	A, B2, Niacin
Ice cream	170	4	7	25	64	B1, B2, Niacin
Margarine	740	–	81	–	16	A
Eggs	150	12	11	–	75	A, B1, B2, Niacin
Pork(Grilled)	340	29	24	–	36	B2, Niacin
Chicken (Roast)	150	25	5	–	55	–
Fish (eg.Cod)	220	20	10	8	60	B1, Niacin
Beans (Boiled)	20	2	–	3	90	A
Cabbage (Boiled)	10	1	–	1	96	A,C
Carrot (Boiled)	20	0.6	–	4	91	A
Cauliflower (Boiled)	10	1.5	–	1	93	C
Cucumber (Boiled)	10	0.6	–	2	96	C
Peas (Boiled)	50	5	–	8	80	A, B1, B2, Niacin, C
Potatoes (Boiled)	80	1	–	22	77	B1
Tomatoes	15	1	–	3	93	A,C
Apples	45	0.3	–	12	84	–

Bananas	80	1	–	20	70	C
Cherries	50	24	–	12	81	–
Grapes	60	0.3	–	15	80	C
Oranges	35	–	–	9	86	C,A
Pea Nuts (Roasted)	570	–	49	9	–	B1, B2, Niacin
Beer	30	–	–	2	–	–
Wine	70	8	–	–	–	–
Spirits	220	2	–	–	–	–
Coffee (Black)	–	6.5	–	–	–	Niacin
Bread	230	6	2	50	39	B1, Niacin
Rice (White Boiled)	120	14	–	30	70	–
Cornflakes with milk	205	–	4	34.7	–	A1, B1, B2, Niacin,B
Chocolate Biscuits	520	–	28	67	2	B2,Niacin
Wheat Bran	200	–	6	23	8	B1, B2, Niacin

CALORIE CHART 2

Dish	Amount	Fat (gms)	Cholestrol (mgs)	Calories (kcals)
Paratha	1 (6")	11	0	180
Puri	1 (4")	5	0	150
Roti	1 (6")	1.5	0	85
Misi Roti	1 (6")	1	0	90
Daal (Urad) with tarka	150gms	6	0	154
Daal (Urad) without tarka	150gms	0.5	0	104
Rajma/Chana/ Lobia	150gms	5	0	153
Dahi/Curd	150gms	3	14	90
Lassi (salty)	200ml	6	3	90
Lassi (sweet)	200ml	6	4	150
Vegetable	150gms	8	0	142
Mixed Vegetable	150gms	21	0	298
Chicken Tikka	6 pieces	20	85	273
Chicken Curry	150gms	36	85	485
Kebabs (Sheekh)	4 pieces	20	100	308
Meat Curry	150gms	35	135	485
Halwa	100gms	15	0	331
Gulabjamun	2 medium	15	31	280

CALORIE CHART 3

Name	Quantity	Calories
Sweets		
Barfi	1pc	100
Halwa	1pc	570
Gulab Jamun	1pc	100
Jalebi	1pc	200
Mysore Pak	1pc	357
Rasgolla	1pc	150
Ladoo	40gms	250
Petha	40gms	250
Balu Shah	40gms	250
Imarti	40gms	250
Patisa	40gms	250
Mesu	40gms	250
Rasmalai	40gms	250
Sohan Halwa	40gms	250
Malpuri	40gms	250

CALORIE CHART 4

Food	Serving Size Ounces	Glycemic Load	Cal/ Serving	High in Typtophan
Chickpea hummus dip	1.1	1	11.6	*
Cantaloupe	4.2	4	24	
Watermelon	4.2	4	24	
Blueberries	3.5	5	26.48	
Strawberries/ raspberries	4.2	1	31.73	
Raw Carrots	2.8	2	32.23	
Pineapple	4.2	6	38.29	
Tomato juice (no added sugar)	8.5	4	42.25	
Lean Meats (Chicken, Turkey)	1.5	0	45	*
Mandarin Orange	4.2	4	48	
Orange	4.2	4	48	
Canned peach in juice	4.2	4	48	
Canned Mandarian segments in juice	4.2	6	48.65	
VB Juice	8.5	4	49.29	
Kiwi	4.2	7	54.56	
Cocoa Via Choc covered almonds	1.1	2	55.44	*
Apricot	4.2	3	58.46	
Skim Milk	8.5	4	66.54	*
Apple	4.2	6	72	
Harshey Smartzone bars	1.8	3	72	
Canned vegetable soup made with water	8.5	5	76.05	
Nestles Quik	8.5	5	80	*
Peanuts	1.8	0	93.49	*
Swiss Cheese	1	0	95	*

1/2 Hard Boiled Egg	2.4	0	105.5	*
Cheddar Cheese	1	0	114.16	*
Gruyere Cheese	1	0	116.95	*
Yoplait Light	7.1	10	117.5	*
Low fat soy milk	8.5	4	126.75	
Roasted and salted mixed nuts	1.8	4	127.49	*
Flavoured mousee	1.8	4	131.21	*
Mixed nuts with raisins	1.8	3	139.71	*
Vanilla or choc instant pudding	3.5	6	153.38	*
Canned baked beans	5.3	6	156.06	*

TABLE 2. GLYCEMIC INDEX FOR SELECTED FOODS (RELATED TO GLUCOSE)

Food	Glycemic index (Glucose = 100)	Serving Size	Carbohydrate per serving (g)
Dates, dried	103	2 oz (60g)	40
Cornflakes	81	1 cup (30g)	26
Jelly beans	78	1 oz (30g)	28
Puffed rice cakes	78	3 cakes (25g)	21
Russet Potato	76	1 medium (150g)	30
Doughnut	76	1 medium (47g)	23
Soda crackers	74	4 crackers (25g)	17
White bread	73	1 large slice (30g)	14
Table sugar (sucrose)	68	2 tsp (10g)	10
Pan cake	67	6" diameter (80g)	58
White Rice (boiled)	64	1 cup (150g)	36
Brown Rice (boiled)	55	1 cup (150g)	36
Spaghetti, white; boiled 10-15 min	44	1 cup (140g)	33
Spaghetti, white; boiled 5 min	38	1 cup (140g)	40
Spaghetti, whole wheat; boiled	37	1 cup (140g)	37
Rye, pumpernickel bread	41	1 large slice (30g)	12
Oranges, raw	42	1 medium (120g)	11
Pears, raw	38	1 medium (120g)	11
Apples, raw	38	1 medium (120g)	15
All-Bran TN cereal	38	1 cup (30g)	23
Skim Milk	32	8 fl oz (250ml)	13
Lentils, dried; boiled	29	1 cup (150g)	18
Kidney beans, dried; boiled	28	1 cup (150g)	25
Pearled barley; boiled	25	1 cup (150g)	42
Cashew nuts	22	1 oz (30g)	9
Peanuts	14	1 oz (30g)	6

NUTRITIVE VALUE OF MILK AND MILK PRODUCTS

	Energy (Kcals)	Moisture (g)	Protein (g)	Fat (g)	Mineral (g)	Fiber (g)	Carbohydrates (g)	Calcium (mg)	Phosphorus (mg)	Iron (mg)
Milk, Buffalo	117	81	4	6	1	-	5	210	130	0
Milk, Cows	67	87	3	4	1	-	4	120	90	0
Milk, goats	72	87	3	4	1	-	5	170	120	0
Milk, human	65	88	1	3	0	-	7	28	11	-
Curds-cows milk	60	89	3	4	1	-	3	149	93	0
Buttermilk	15	97	1	1	0	-	0	30	30	0
Skimmed milk, liquid	29	92	2	0	2	-	5	120	90	0
Channa, cows milk	265	57	18	21	3	-	1	208	138	-
Channa, Buffalo milk	292	54	13	23	2	-	8	480	277	-
Cheese	348	40	24	25	4	-	6	790	520	2
Khoa whole buffalo milk	421	31	15	31	3	-	20	650	420	6
Khoa skimmed milk	206	46	22	2	4	-	26	990	650	3
Khoa, whole cow milk	413	25	20	26	4	-	25	956	613	-
Skimmed milk powder	357	4	38	0	7	-	51	1370	1000	1
Whole milk powder	496	3	26	27	6	-	38	950	730	1

CALORIE EXPENDITURE CHART

Activity Done for 30 Minutes at:	Calories Burned per 30 Minutes of Activity at your weight										
	100lbs	120 lbs	140lbs	160lbs	180lbs	200lbs	220lbs	240lbs	260lbs	280lbs
Aerobic Dancing	115	138	161	184	207	230	253	276	299	322
Aerobic Step Training	145	174	203	232	261	290	319	348	377	406
Backpacking (20 lb load)	200	240	280	320	360	400	440	480	520	560
Basketball	130	156	182	208	234	260	286	312	338	364
Bicycling	200	240	280	320	360	400	440	480	520	560
Dancing	100	120	140	160	180	200	220	240	260	280
Gardening	90	108	126	144	162	180	198	216	234	252
Golf walking without cart	100	120	140	160	180	200	220	240	260	280
Housework	90	108	126	144	162	180	198	216	234	262
Jogging (5 mph)	185	222	259	296	333	370	407	444	481	518
Mowing	135	162	189	216	243	270	297	324	351	378
Skipping Rope	285	342	399	456	513	570	627	684	741	798
Stair Climber Machine	160	192	224	256	288	320	352	384	416	448
Swimming (25yards per min)	120	144	168	192	216	240	264	288	312	336
Walking (15minute mile)	100	120	140	160	180	200	220	240	260	280
Weight Training (90secs between sets)	125	150	175	200	225	250	275	300	325	350

SAMPLE DIET CHARTS

BALANCED DIET

Name	Mr XYZ	BMR(Lean)			Diet type	Low carb (25:45:30)
Age	30years	TEE	Kcal/day		Carbs	100
Weight	91kg	Calorie deficit	Kcal/day		Proteins	180
Height	171cm	Calorie target	Kcal/day		Fats	53
Lean Weight	70kgs	Protein target	lean mass*1.8gm	156		
Body Fat %	28%					

Time	Food Item	Qnty	Carbs(gms)	Protein(gms)	Fats(gms)	Calories	Additional Remarks
Upon waking up	Luke warm water with lemon	1 cup	-			2	
Breakfast (9am)	Boiled eggs(egg white)	5		20	0	85	Fiber 4 gms
						0	
						0	

11.30 noon	Green tea	1 cup				0	
	Almonds, walnuts, cashew, pistachio mix	28 (gms)	4	6	17	193	
Lunch (2pm)	Plain wheat roti	1 pc	17	3	1	91	Fibre_2.7gms
	Chick peas/ kedney beans	80gms	9	3	1	54	Fibre_3gms
	Green veggies boiled	100gms				0	Fibre_2.7gms
	Onion cucumber cabbage tomato salad	100gms				0	Just before lunch
Pre workout (4pm)	Boiled Chana	60gms	17	5	2	102	
	Peanuts	15gms	2	4	7	92	
	Onion, tomato, cucumber	25gms					

Workout (5:30pm)							
Past workout (7pm)	Whey protein	1scoop	4	24	2	130	Fiber 2gms
	Apple	1pc	21	0	1	93	Fibre 5gms
Dinner	Plain wheat roti	1pc	17	3	1	91	Fibre_2.7gms
	Paneer Bhurji	150gms	5	16	21	274	Fibre_1.2gms
	Total		96	83	53	1205	
	Target		100	180	53	0	
	Deficit/(excess)		4	97	_0	_1205	
	Target Protein as per lean mass		156				

	24(180_156) gms		To be adjusted with carbs
Diff between lean and full mass target			
Revised macros target	Target(gms)	As per chart	Deficit/(excess)
Carbs	124	96	28
Protein	156	83	73
Fats	53	53	_0

VEGETARIAN DIET CHART 1

Age-29

Weight-70

Height-5ft, 4

Food item	Quantity	Fats(g)	Carbs(g)	Protein(g)	Calories
Upon waking up					
Warm water+lime	1glass	0	0	0	0
Breakfast					
Amul cheese slice/cube	2	13	0.6	10	159.4
Almond	10	6.8	2.37	2.55	80.88
Spinach/any other green leafy vegetable	100g				
Lunch					
Paneer	100g	20	0	18	252
Cucumber	100g	0.1	3.6	0.7	18.1
Walnut	40g	26.08	5.48	6.09	281
Ghee/Butter/Coconut oil/Olive oil	5g	5	0	0	45
Snack					
Amul cheese slice/cube	2	13	0.6	10	159.4
Almond	10	6.8	2.37	2.55	80.88
Spinach/any other green leafy vegetable	100g				
Dinner (1-2 hours before sleep)					
Paneer	100g	20	0	18	252
Cucumber	100g	0.1	3.6	0.7	18.1
Walnut	40g	26.08	5.48	6.09	281
Ghee/Butter/Coconut oil/Olive oil	5g	5	0	0	45
Total Macros		141.96	24.1	74.68	1672.76

VEGETARIAN DIET CHART 2

Age-41   Weight-57   Height-   Fat-   BMR-1120
                            165cm   26.74%   TEE-
                                                1344.66

FOOD ITEM		QTY	F(g)	P(g)	C(g)
Warm water+ACV					
Green tea					
Green smoothie					
Pre & post Workout					
Black coffee					
Whey protein	scoop	1	1	25	2
Breakfast					
Paneer	gms	50	10.5	9	1
Lunch					
Paneer	gms	150	31.5	27	3
Ghee	gms	5	5	0	0
Spinach	gms	100			
Cucumber	no.	1			
Snacks					
Whey protein	scoop	1	1	25	2
Cabbage	gms	100			
Dinner					
Paneer	gms	100	21	18	2
Ghee	gms	10	10	0	0
Spinach	gms	100			
TOTAL MACROS			80	104	10
MACROS NEEDED			80	105	15

VEGETARIAN DIET CHART FOR FEMALES

Mrs XYZ

BMR	1255	Weight	60kg		
TEE	1506	Height	152cms		
BODY FAT%	26.38%				
Target Calories	1300				
Macros		Carbs	Protein	Fats	Calories
		81.25	113.75	57.78	1300
Upon waking up (7am)					
Almonds	5	1.18	1.28	3.04	35
Black coffee/Black tea	200ml	0	0	0	1
Breakfast (9am)					
Green veggies	100gm				
Whey protein	1 scoop	4	24	2	130
Onion/Tomato/ Cucumber					
Lunch (1pm)					
Paneer	100gm	25	1	25	170
Coconutoil/butter/ ghee/canola	10ml			4	35
Green veggies	100gm				
Rice	50gm	5	40	2	170
Curd	1cup(100gms)	3.45	11.75	4.2	100
Onion/Tomato/ Cucumber					
Evening Snacks (5pm)					
Black coffee					1
Dinner (8.30pm)					
Paneer	100gm	25	1	25	170
Coconutoil/butter/ ghee/canola	10ml			10	90
Rice	50gm	5	40	2	170
Total		67.45	117.75	74.2	1204

Target		81.25	113.75	57.78	1300
Difference		13.8	-4	-16.42	96

Makhana	50 gms	37	5	0	180

VEGETARIAN DIET CHART FOR MALES

Mr XYZ

BMR	1774	Weight	97kg		
TEE	2129.6	Height	172cms		
Target Calories	1700				
Macros		Carbs	Protein	Fats	Calories
		81.25	113.75	57.78	1300
Upon waking up (7am)					
Almonds	5	1.18	1.28	3.04	35
Black coffee/Black tea	200ml	0	0	0	1
Breakfast (9am)					
Green veggies	100gm				0
Whey protein	1 scoop	4	24	2	130
Onion/Tomato/Cucumber					
Lunch (1pm)					
Paneer	100gm	0	23	27	338
Rice	10ml	27.9	2.66	0.28	129
Curd	1cup (100gms)	3.45	11.75	4.2	100
Ghee/Butter/Coconut oil	10gms			10	90
Onion/Tomato/Cucumber	100gm				
Evening Snacks (5pm)					
Black coffee					1
Dinner (8.30pm)					
Soya Chunks	100gm	20	52	2	306
Ghee/Butter/Coconut oil	10gms			10	90
Curd	1cup (100gms)	3.45	11.75	4.2	100
Green veggies	100gms				
Rice	50gms	14	1	0	65
Total		73.98	127.44	62.72	1385

Target		106	149	75	1700
Difference		32.02	21.56	12.28	315

Makhana	50 gms	37	5	0	180

LOW CALORIE DIET CHART 1

	Quantity	Fats	Carbs	Protein	Calories
Weight	113				
Body fat	31.00%				
BMR	2060				
Goal	Fat loss				
Tee	2845.47				
Low carb diet macros(25:35:40)		127	178	249	
	Quantity	Fats	Carbs	Protein	Calories
Breakfast - 9 am					
Boiled egg without yolk	5	0	1	20	86
Almonds	5	3.05	1.2	1.3	35
Milk	100ml	3	5	3	58
Museli, kolloggs Extra Museli - Nuts Delight	40gm	2	36	6	180
Guava - 11am	1 medium	1	13	2	61
Lunch - 1pm					
Paneer	100gm	21	3	9	277
Tomato	1 small	0.25	4.8	1.82	22
Onion	1 medium	0.1	11	1	44
1 tbsp oil		13	0	0	120
Broccoli	100 gm	0.3	7	3	34
1 chapati		3	20	4	120
Amul Chach	2	2	0	4	52
Pre workout - 4pm					
Almonds	5	3.05	1.2	1.3	35

Green Tea - at 6pm	1 cup				
Dinner - 9 pm					
Paneer	100gm	21	3	9	277
Tomato	1 small	0.25	4.8	1.82	22
Onion	1 medium	0.1	11	1	44
1 tbsp oil		13	0	0	120
Broccoli	100 gm	0.3	7	3	34
1 chapati		3	20	4	120
Milk - 10:30 pm	100ml	3	5	3	58
Total		92.4	154	78.24	1799

LOW CALORIE DIET CHART 2

Food Item	Quantity	Fats(gms)	Carbs(gms)	Protein(gms)	Calories	Additional Instructions
Upon Waking up						
1 glass luke warm water + lemon (no sugars)						Vitamin C 1 tab 500mg+1 multivitamin (any) +
Post workout						
1 scoop whey	1 Scoop	2.4	1.5	24	120	
Breakfast						
2 whole egg	2	9.94	0.76	12.58	148	
1 teaspoon butter	1	4	0	0	40	
1 cube cheese - cheddar	1	6.4	0	4.8	77	
Lunch						
Dal	15g	0.1	9	3.9	53	
200 grms Chicken Breast	200	8	0	48	264	

1 medium onion (100grms)	1	0	10	0.9	44	
1 medium tomato (100 grms)	1	0.2	3.9	0.9	18	
200 grms spinach / broccoli/ cabbage	200					Have 1 tbsp of Isabgol/ psyllium husk with water
1 teaspoon ghee	1	5	0	0	50	
1 cup curd (home made Indian)	1 cup	4	0	3	60	
Dinner (1-2 hours before sleep)						
60 grms rice	60g	0	49.3	4	213	
1 teaspoon ghee	1	5	0	0	50	
100 grms paneer	100	20.8	1.25	18.4	265	
Bellpepper (50g)	50g	0.1	2.3	0.45	10	
Total Macros		65.94	78.01	120.93	1412	
Target Macros		62.2	87.5	122.5	1400	

LOW CALORIE DIET CHART 3

	Age - 28					
	Sex - Female					
	Weight - 65 kgs					
	Height - 5'4"					
	Fat % - 30.9					
	BMR = 1321.15					
	TEE = 2278.98					
	Diet - LCD (25C:35P:40F)					
	C - 82.63g P-115.67g F-58.76g					
Time	Food Item	Quantity	Calories	Fat (g)	Carb (g)	Protein (g)
	Upon waking up					
08:30	Water + ACV	1 litre + 1 tsp	0	0	0	0
09:00	Apple	Half	44	0.4	9.9	0.2
10:15 to 11:15 AM	Yoga					
	Post Yoga					
11:30	Whey	1 Scoop (30g)	117	1	2	25
	Breakfast					
12:00	Egg Whites	4	69	0.2	1	14.4
	Oats Chila	40g oats	156	2.8	26.5	6.8
	Onion	1	32	0.1	7.5	0.9
	Ghee	1 tbsp	135	15	0	0
13:00	Green Tea	1	0	0	0	0
	Lunch					
15:00	Egg Whites	4	69	0.2	1	14.4
	Capsicum	1	18	0.2	3.2	1
	Cucumber	1	16	0.1	3.1	0.5
	Tomato	1	12	0.1	2.2	1.1
	Garlic	6 cloves	27	0.1	6	1.2

	Paneer	50 g	133	10.4	0.6	9.2
	Ghee	1/2 tbsp	67.5	7.5	0	0
16:30	Spinach	100 g	0	0	0	0
5:00 to 7:00 PM	Pre Workout					
	Black Coffee	1	0	0	0	0
19:30	Gym					
	Post Workout					
	Whey	1 Scoop (30g)	120	1	2	25
21:30	Dinner					
	Paneer	50 g	133	10.4	0.6	9.2
23:30	Rice (steamed without starch)	100g	115	0.3	25.6	2.5
	Curd	100g	60	3	4.4	3.2
	Green coffee	1	0	0	0	0
	Total Macros		1323.5	52.8	95.6	114.6
	IDEAL Macros		1321.5	58.76	82.63	115.67

LOW CALORIE DIET CHART 4

Age	35				
Height	178				
Weight	99 kgs				
Fat %	31				
BMR	1816				
TEE	2179				
Starting Cal	1800				
Meals	**Contents**	**Protein(Grams)**	**Fat (Grams)**	**Carbs (Grams)**	**Calories**
Whey	1 Scoop	28.5	0	0	122
Brekfast					
Green Veggies	100grms	1		1	7
Paneer	50gm	9	10.5	0.75	132
Brunch					
Curd	200gm	24	8.6	7	210
Lunch					
Paneer	100gm	18	21	1.5	265
Ghee / Coconut oil / butter	14gm		14		124
Spinach	1 Cup	1		1	7
Peanuts	50gm	14	26	7.2	299
Evening					
Almonds	10	5	1.8	2.5	62.2
Cheese Slice	1 slice	4	5	0.5	62
Whey	1 Scoop	28.5	0	0	122
Dinner					
Spinach	1 Cup	1		1	7
Paneer	100gm	18	21	1.5	265

Ghee / Coconut oil / butter	14gm		14		124
TOTAL		**152**	**121.9**	**23.95**	**1808.2**

LOW CARB DIET CHART

Mr XYZ	Target Calories				
Weight	77kg				
Height	178cm				
BMR	1750 cal				
Meal	Food Item	Quantity	Carbs (25%)	Protein (35%)	Fats (45%)
Morning	Lemon in luke warm water	1 Lemon	4	0	0
Breakfast	Omellete	2 eggs	1	12	10
	Butter	5gm	0	0	4
	Whey	1 Scoop	3	25	2
Lunch	Panner	100gm	5	20	20
	Butter	5gm	0	0	4
	Curd	100gm	5.5	16	6
Snacks	Boiled Eggs	4 eggs	1.5	24	20
PosT Workout	Whey	1 scoop	3	25	2
Dinner	Rice Uncooked	40gm	32	3	0
	Onion	50gm	5	0	0
	Tomato	50gm	2	0	0
	Lentils uncooked	50gm	30	13	0
	Oil	10gm	0	0	9
	Soya Chunks Uncooked	20g	6	10	0
Total Macros			98	148	77
Calories			392	592	693
Net Calories		1677	23	35	41

KETO DIET 1

Name:Mrs XYZ									
Age:30yrs	BMR:1371.4Kcal per day								
Weight:74kgs	TEE:1645.68Kcal per day				Exer:walk for an hour(brisk+normal)				
Height:5'2"	Carbs:17.14 gm				& home exercise & stretching				
	Proteins:120 gm				Water:3ltrs per day approx				
BF%:25	Fats:92 gm								
Ingredient/Item	Fat(g)	Protein(g)	Carbs(g)	Calories	Servings	Fat(g)	Protein(g)	Net carbs(g)	Calories
Breakfast									
Cheese slice	5	4	0	113	2	10	8	0	226
Whole Egg	5	6	1	74	2	10	12	2	148
Almonds	0.6	0.3	0.3	7	2	1.2	0.6	0.6	14
11:00 AM									
Egg whites	0.1	3.6	0.2	17	2	0.2	7.2	0.4	34
Almond	0.6	0.3	0.3	7	2	1.2	0.6	0.6	14

93

Lunch										
Chicken boneless	2.6	31	0	151	1		2.6	31	0	151
Ghee/butter/oil	20	0	0	180	1		20	0	0	180
Whole eggs	5	6	1	74	2		10	12	2	148
Snack										
Black coffee+coconut oil										
1 TSP(15gm)	15	0	0		1		15	0	0	0
Whey protein										
Scoop	1	25	4	100	1		1	25	4	100
Dinner										
Chicken boneless	2.6	31	0	151	1		2.6	31	0	151
Broccoli	0	0.03	0.07	0.34	100		0.4	2.95	7	34
Ghee/butter/Oil	20	0	0	180	1		20	0	0	180
Totals							94.2	130.35	16.6	1380

KETO DIET 2

Time	Qnty	Weight=64kg		Height=156 cms		BMR=1413.9	Required calories=1700	
		Proteins gms	Carbs gms	Fats gms	Calories gms	Required calories-1700	Proteins=191	45%
6.ooam								
Lemon water	1 glass						Carbs=106	25%
Breakfast								
Oil/ghee	10ml	0	0	10	85		Fats=57	30%
Chole salad	1bowl	14.5	7.9	4.2	268			
Paneer	50gms	9	0.6	10	132			
Morning snacks								
Almonds	10	2	2.5	5	35			

95

Lunch							
Soya chunks	75gm	39	24	0	260		
Egg whites	6	21.6	1.4	0.3	103		
Eve snacks							
Almonds	10	2	2.5	5	35		
Chana sprouts with spinach	50gms	9	30	3	182		
Cheese cube	1	5		7	80		
Post/pre workout							
Whey protein	2scoops	50	6	4	240		
Dinner							
Soya chunks	75gm	39	24	0	260		
Oil/ghee	10ml	0	0	10	85		
Total Macros		191.1	98.9	59	1765		

KETO DIET 3

Age	32	Weight	60kgs	Height	5ft 2in	BMR	1321
Food Item	Time	Quantity	Carbs	Protein	Fat	Calories	
Pre workout	6						
Lemon+Warm water			0	0	0	0	
Post workout	7.15						
Soaked almonds		5	2	2	3	35	ACV 1 Tpsn
Boiled eggs		4	0	28	20	280	1 multivitamin
Mid day snacks	10.00						
Cheese slice		1	0	4	5	62	
Lunch	14.00						
Paneer		100 gms	2	20	20	250	
Green veggies		100 gms					
Evening snacks	17.00						
Green tea							
Almonds		5	2	2	3	35	
Dinner	20.00						
Boiled eggs		4	0	28	20	280	
Paneer		100 gms	2	20	20	250	
Green veggies		200 gms					
Ghee		20 ml	0	0	20	180	

KETO DIET 4

Name	XYZ (male)	BMR	1500	Height	5'10"	Diet Tenure	6 weeks
Weight	93kgs	TEE	2000	Diet Type	Keto	Week	1st week
Meal	Food Item	Qnty	Unit	Sum of carb	Sum of fat	Sum of Protein	Sum of calories
Breakfast	Cheese slice	1.00	piece	0.3	5.00	4.00	62.00
	Egg	2.00	piece		9.00	14.00	160.00
	Ghee	5.00	gm		5.00		43.00
	Whey	15.00	gm	0.6	0.5	12.5	60.00
Breakfast Total				0.9	19.5	30.5	325.00
Lunch	Coconut oil	5.00	gm		5.0		43.00
	Cucumber	80.00	gm	2		0.56	11.84
	Onion	10.00	gm	0.75	0.01	0.11	4.00
	Paneer	100.00	gm	3.3	23.3	20.0	300
	Tomato	30.00	gm	0.81	0.06	0.27	5.4
	Spinach	100.00	gm				
Lunch Total				6.86	28.37	20.94	364.24
Post work out	Almond	7.00	piece	0.7	4.2	2.1	49.00
	Whey	30.00	gm	1.2	1.00	25	120.00
Post workout Total				1.9	5.2	27.1	169.00
Evening	Egg white	4.00	piece			14.00	56.00
Evening Total						14.00	56.00
Dinner	Capsicum	20.00	gm	0.26		0.2	3.2
	Curd	100.00	gm	4.4	3.1	4.00	62.00
	Ghee	5.00	gm		5		43.00
	Onion	10.00	gm	0.75	0.01	0.11	4.00
	Paneer	150.00	gm	4.95	34.95	30	450.00
	Tomato	30.00	gm	0.81	0.06	0.27	5.4

Dinner Total				11.17	43.12	34.58	567.6
Grand Total				20.83	96.19	127.12	1481.84
Calories				83.32	865.71	508.48	1481.84
Macro %				5.62	58.42	34.31	100.00